Routine
Complications

Routine Complications

Troubles with Talk between Doctors and Patients

CANDACE WEST

INDIANA UNIVERSITY PRESS

BLOOMINGTON

Copyright © 1984 by Candace West
Manufactured in the United States of America

Library of Congress Cataloging in Publication Data

West, Candace.
    Routine complications.

    Bibliography: p.
    Includes index.
    1. Physician and patient. 2. Interpersonal
communication. I. Title. [DNLM: 1. Physician-
patient relations. 2. Communication. W 62 W516r]
R727.3.W44 1984   610.69'6   83-48733
ISBN 0-253-35030-1
1 2 3 4 5 88 87 86 85 84

For Gilly West, M.A., P.N.P.
and James R. West, M.D.

Contents

Tables

Acknowledgments

No book is written alone, no matter how sole the
authorship.
—Nancy Henley, *Body Politics*

The pages that follow this one are populated by the ghosts of a
great many friends and colleagues. From beginning to end, I enjoyed
the benefits of a larger community than obtains between a book and
its author.

My initial idea for this project was inspired by a series of exciting
discussions with Arlene Daniels, Nancy Henley, and Virginia Oleson.
I am greatly indebted to them for sharing my early enthusiasm for
the research and especially for helping me to sustain it through their
insights, challenges, and gentle corrections.

Implementation of the study would not have been possible without
the help of Al Bayer, Al Imershein, Bob Pantell, and Tom Stewart.
Collectively, they offered invaluable assistance in securing access to
my research setting; individually, they provided many careful
criticisms of my ideas.

For raising questions I did not want to ask and helping me to find
answers to them, I am most grateful to Sarah F. Berk, Paul Ekman,
the late Erving Goffman, Judy Martin, Ann Stromberg, Tom Wilson,
and Don Zimmerman. My preliminary analyses were greatly
strengthened by the queries they posed and new ones were prompted
by their suggestions.

Rich Frankel, Wendy Martyna, Barrie Thorne, and Gilly West were
indispensable to me in this venture. For long hours of detailed
discussions, innumerable insightful additions to my ideas and
unstinting encouragement, I owe them more than I can say.

Linda Guiffre and Sofia Gruskin worked long hours as research
assistants during the early stages of investigation, helping to type,
code, and analyze hundreds of pages of transcribed interaction.
Although Angela Garcia joined me in the final stages of production,
her contributions were no less impressive—making long trips to
medical libraries, poring through the endless details of bibliographic
references, and availing me of her superb editorial skills on the final

draft. Jan Burton labored as my manuscript editor and moral supporter during earlier drafts, and Lyn Smith typed and retyped these pages more times than either of us can remember.

For financial support for this research, I am grateful to the Southern Regional Educational Board, the Committee on Research and Junior Faculty Development Committee at the University of California, Santa Cruz, and the Organized Research Unit in Institutional Analysis and Social Policy at Santa Cruz, directed by Bob Alford. The generous assistance of these agencies provided for my travel and subsistence during early stages of data collection, the wherewithal to analyze the data, and, most important, the release time I needed to devote my energies to research.

In writing this book, I have incurred considerable intellectual debts. Those most outstanding are owed to the late Erving Goffman, Nancy Henley, the late Harvey Sacks, Emanuel Schegloff, and, especially, Gail Jefferson. Of course, none of them is responsible for my mistakes and deficiencies.

Personal debts have also piled up, particularly with Dane Archer, Pam Roby, Sharon Veach, and Stephen Williams. The suggestions and encouragement of these cheer leaders carried me through many a low period.

Finally, I offer my heartfelt thanks and appreciation to the patients, residents, and staff of the Department of Family Medicine, Medical University of South Carolina in Charleston. I hope that this work will be of some use to them in their work and thus will help to reimburse them for what I owe.

Candace West

Santa Cruz, California, January 1984

Transcribing Conventions Used in the Text

The transcript techniques and symbols were devised by Gail Jefferson in the course of research undertaken with Harvey Sacks. Techniques are revised, symbols added or dropped as they seem useful to work. There is no guarantee or suggestion that the symbols or transcripts alone would permit the doing of any unspecified research tasks: They are properly used as an adjunct to the tape-recorded materials.

Mary: I don' ⎡know⎤ John ⎣you⎦ don't	Brackets indicate that the portions of utterances so encased are simultaneous. The left-hand bracket marks the onset of simultaneity, the right-hand bracket indicates its resolution.
A: We:::ll now	Colons indicate that the immediately prior syllable is prolonged.
A: But-	A hyphen represents a cutting off short of the immediately prior syllable.
CAPS or <u>underscoring</u>	Both of these are used to represent heavier emphasis (in speaker's pitch) on words so marked.
A: Swat I said = B: = But you didn't	Equal signs are used to indicate that no time elapsed between the objects "latched" by the marks. Often used as a transcribing convenience, they can also mean that a next speaker starts at precisely the end of a current speaker's utterance.
(1.3)	Numbers encased in parentheses indicate the seconds and tenths of seconds ensuing between speaker turns. They may also be used to indicate the duration of pauses internal to a speaker's turn.

(#) — Score sign indicates a pause of about a second that it wasn't possible to discriminate precisely.

(word) — Single parentheses with words in them indicate that something was heard, but the transcriber is not sure what it was. These can serve as a warning that the transcript may be unreliable.

((softly)) — Double parentheses enclose "descriptions" not transcribed utterances.

A: I (x) I did — Parentheses encasing an "x" indicate a hitch or stutter on the part of the speaker.

A: Oh Yeah? — Punctuation marks are used for intonation, not grammar.

( ) — Empty parentheses signify untimed pauses.

°So you did. — The degree symbol represents softness, or decreased amplitude.

.hh, hh, eh-heh, .engh-henh — These are breathing and laughing indicators. A period followed by "hh's" marks an inhalation. The "hh's" alone stand for exhalation. The "eh-heh" and ".engh-henh" are laughter syllables (inhaled when preceded by a period).

(.) — The period encased in parentheses denotes a pause of one tenth of a second.

Routine
Complications

CHAPTER 1

Troubles with Talk between Doctors and Patients

An increasing number of lay and scholarly sources have suggested that something is "wrong" with the talk that goes on between patients and their doctors. Medical journals, popular magazines, and scientific periodicals are rife with advice on what to do about it.

From a physician's perspective, the issue is in part one of medical management: the need for more efficient use of time, energy, and money. Fischl (1976), for example, argues that patient dissatisfaction with health care would "simmer down considerably" if physicians would only spell out the procedures they employ in treatment and diagnosis. "Show and tell," he urges, and "Don't be too modest to claim credit when things go right" (pp. 231–236). His suggestion is typical of a body of literature which identifies significant ties between practitioners' practical concerns (e.g., time and money) on the one hand, and their communication with patients on the other (see Davis, 1978; Lavin, 1977; Rosenberg, 1977; and Siegel, 1977, for illustrative instances). Admittedly, many practicing physicians see a conflict between the two. Dr. Manuel Rowen titles one article "Do you always hear out your patients? I don't" (1977). As he explains: "I confess! I'm guilty! I *often* cut the patient short, and I expect to keep right on doing so. It's the only way I can stay in practice. I simply have to preserve my emotional, physical and mental energies if I'm to perform my job" (Rowen, 1977:82). From Rowen's perspective, it would appear that the day-to-day demands of practicing medicine may preclude a two-way flow of communication between physicians and patients. Talk, in short, is not cheap.

1

For one thing, talking with patients takes time—and time is a precious resource in "Medical Economics." In a medical magazine of the same title, physician Mostyn Davis confides: "In the early days of my practice, I used to sit down with a patient and take the history face to face. That wasted a lot of my time. . . . Today I use a form that patients can fill out themselves, largely by circling Yes or No answers. This is not only a time-saver—it also gives patients the feeling that they are contributing to their own care" (*Medical Economics*, 1978:95). Whether or not Davis' patients actually feel a greater sense of participation in their care while circling those Yeses and Noes, he is probably correct in assuming that face-to-face interaction takes more time.

Face-to-face with their patients, physicians may need not only to spend more time eliciting responses from them, but also to spend time replying to their patients' interrogations. Dr. Irwin M. Siegel puts forth a tongue-in-cheek view of just such a predicament:

> "Doctor, I have this short list of questions I've written down. It won't take but a minute."
> The French have a name for it, "le malade avec le petit papier" (the patient with the little paper). She suffered the malady in both its acute and chronic forms.
> "I suppose you think these are foolish questions?"
> Tiny, molelike, a 68-year-old former high school teacher.
> "I saw this television program last night, all about leukemia. One of the symptoms was fatigue. I often get tired. Do you think I have leukemia?"
> "No, I don't think you have leukemia; your fatigue is natural for your age."
> "Well, that's certainly a relief. Now, how about exercise? Do you think I get enough exercise?"
> "As I told you last visit. . . ." (1977:149)

Because she is stereotyped, Siegel's "tiny, molelike" interrogator is perhaps intended to be amusing.

But Dr. John Fisher warns of a more serious threat associated with patient questions: "A little learning is not only a dangerous thing. When exhibited by patients, it can also be downright annoying. And more and more patients are exhibiting it. With the growing number of pseudoscientific articles in the lay press, the physician's word is increasingly being questioned" (1977:169). Fisher seems to imply that the very legitimacy of the physician's occupational status may be imperiled by patients' growing inquisitiveness.

Although many physicians may share Fisher's concerns for the consequences of increased patient assertiveness, they are also likely to shudder at the thought of shouldering total responsibility for patients' health. Especially in these times, when the costs of playing God are high, doctors are prone to welcome patient education programs which spread the obligation of responsibile health-related communication over their relationships with patients. Serious long-term difficulties can arise from "failures to communicate," including ambiguities whose resolution is likely to take place in the courtroom (cf. Veatch, 1977; Neumann, 1977).

Ironically, as Horsley and Lavin (1977) point out, the courtroom is precisely the place in which what you tell a patient and what you ask a patient will count most. In avoiding potential malpractice charges, for example:

> I believe a doctor can avoid statistics as much as possible in discussing risks and still protect himself. You can say, "In a very small number of cases, this or that complication may occur. I've never had such a complication in my experience, and neither have any of the other doctors I know. But it is cited in the medical literature on this operation."
>
> To me, such a statement to the patient makes the situation far clearer than talk about a "point five per cent risk" of something or other, which the Puerto Rican patient . . . for instance, certainly isn't going to understand anyway. Nor will the average housewife or assembly-line worker or whoever. (Horsley and Lavin, 1977:154)

Clearly, Horsley and Lavin's suggestions reflect a relatively poor opinion of patients' abilities—at least those of patients whose ethnicity, gender, or occupational status differs from that of most physicians. Thus, the doctor "informing" the potential hysterectomy patient is advised to use such expressions as "very small" or "one patient in a thousand" when discussing the risks of her surgery.

Should that doctor end up in a courtroom, however, much more precise language will be required. Dr. Leonard Berlin warns physicians that speaking in generalities can actually contribute to successful prosecution of malpractice cases:

> Terms like "may be," or "perhaps," or "not completely diagnostic," or "cannot be excluded" may help another doctor in making a diagnosis, but they don't belong in expert-witness statements.

The result too often is that an expert witness is dismayed to find later that his statement—supposedly concluding that no wrong has been committed—is being used against an innocent doctor. It is giving the plaintiff's attorney bargaining power. It is even safeguarding the attorney against countersuit by giving him "reasonable cause" to act. (1977:121)

Be specific, then, when speaking with other professionals, but stick to generalities when talking with patients?

PATIENTS' PERSPECTIVES

The physician who attempts to follow such advice is likely to run into difficulties. Increasingly, even popular magazines devote a good deal of monthly space to advising potential patients on how they can pin down problems involved with talking to their doctors. Most "women's" magazines have traditionally featured regular columns on health care, even though they are sometimes hidden in the "Beauty" sections (e.g., *Glamour* or *Vogue*). Recently, however, entire articles have been devoted to medical communication. *Family Circle*, for example, offered readers "How to Understand Your Doctor" through an alphabetized "Guide to Medical Language" (Nierenberg and Janovic, 1979). *Cosmopolitan* featured "Are You a Smart Patient?" (Belsky, 1978), stressing important questions patients often forget to ask. Another lead article in *Family Circle* (Galton, 1979) specified a dozen or more "Mystery Ailments" potential patients can look for and call to their doctors' attention.

The form, as well as the content, of physician-patient communication, is seen as problematic. In June 1977, the *Los Angeles Times* reported that classes were being offered to physicians which taught translation of medical terminology into language plain enough for patients to understand (Chriss, 1977). By November 1980, Kaiser/Permanente Medical Care Program had hired a college business teacher to instruct physicians in the art of legible writing (e.g., so that prescriptions and post-examination instructions written by physicians might be deciphered by their addressees). Substantial enrollments in both courses indicate the extent to which a doctor-patient communication gap is generally acknowledged.[1]

In short, a "special" (albeit unspecified) sort of communication is generally assumed to characterize the physician-patient relationship. Medical management journals reflect this assumption, devoting a voluminous literature to methods of achieving rapport with patients, strategies for ensuring patients' expression of problems, and devices for ascertaining that physicians' instructions are heard and understood. Popular magazines rely on this assumption in offering advice to potential patients (e.g., how to ask the right questions, how to listen to physicians' instructions, and how to tell what information might assist a physician in making diagnoses).

A major problem with all of these suggestions is their lack of grounding in systematic empirical research. In order to know, for example, how to educate patients to ask "better" questions, one would first want to know what kinds of questions patients can and do ask. Similarly, in educating physicians to "improve" their rapport with patients, one would benefit by knowledge of the kind of rapport which is currently in existence. If better communication is the issue here, then an empirical investigation of the structure of communication itself would surely be a first priority.

SOCIAL SCIENCE AND MEDICINE

Unfortunately, social science has not yet contributed many answers to questions pertaining to medical dialogues, since existing research has not yet addressed the organization of interaction between doctors and patients as a topic in its own right. To be sure, the doctor-patient *relationship* has received considerable sociological attention—more, perhaps, than any other aspect of medicine. We have learned a great deal about the social roles of physician and patient (e.g., Parsons and Fox, 1952), about the profession of doctoring (e.g., Becker et al., 1961; Bucher and Stelling, 1969; Freidson, 1961; 1970a; 1970b; 1975; and Hughes, 1971), and about the distinctive characteristics of social relations between practitioners and patients (e.g., the essential asymmetry of the doctor-patient relationship [cf. Parsons, 1975], the inequality of physicians' and patients' knowledge bases [cf. Hughes, 1971], and the differential standing of doctor and patient vis-à-vis their expert and lay statuses [cf. Freidson, 1970a].) However, the social science of medicine has tended to treat interaction between doctors and patients as a resource for its formulations rather than as an object of inquiry (see Chapter 2). Consequently, doctor-patient communication is often invoked to explain various behavioral outcomes (such as maintenance of professional detachment, acquisition of the social roles of physician and patient, or definition of problematic aspects of social conduct), but it is rarely studied as a form of behavior unto itself.

WOMEN AND HEALTH

Certainly, one important challenge to traditional studies of physician-patient communication derives from feminist analyses of women's relationship to organized medicine (e.g., Corea, 1978; Dreifus, 1977; Ehrenreich and English, 1978; Fee, 1975; Gordon, 1976; Ruzek, 1979; Scully, 1980; Stromberg, forthcoming; and Walsh, 1977). Historical studies trace the loss of women's control over their own bodies to the emergence of medicine as a male-dominated profession (Ehrenreich and English, 1978; Gordon, 1976; Walsh, 1977; and Wertz and Wertz, 1977). Contemporary investigations focus on the implications of this lack of control for such issues as abortion (Luker, 1975; 1984), birthing practices (Arms, 1975; Shaw, 1974), contraception (Corea, 1978; Fisher and Todd, 1983a; Seaman, 1969; Seaman and Seaman, 1977), and surgical intervention (Dreifus, 1977; and Scully, 1980).

Although much of the research on women and health has focused on women's experiences as health care consumers or health care providers, the interactional aspects of their experiences have not gone unnoticed (see Fisher and Todd, 1983b: 9–10, for a general overview of feminist contributions to the field). In seriously attending to women's "personal problems" in interactions with doctors, feminist analyses have revealed the profoundly political dimensions of such encounters:

> Feminists were and are bitter that they are often ignorant not out of choice or inability to understand but because doctors make it difficult to acquire the information they need to make competent decisions for themselves. In waiting rooms, there is little health education material to help patients understand their bodies or aid them in communicating with doctors. In the examining room, they feel demeaned when called "honey" or "dear." Most wonder why they must address physicians as "Doctor X" when they are addressed so familiarly by pseudo-intimate terms or by their first names. Women also complain that when they are stripped and draped and lying on their backs with feet in stirrups, it is difficult to interact with physicians. In such an awkward position,

women can neither see what is being done nor ask questions easily. (Ruzek, 1979:33–34)

As Ruzek observes, feminists' concerns for equality and individual rights to self-determination are thwarted by the mystique surrounding medical interaction rituals (see especially pp. 113–124).

To the extent that relations between doctors and patients tell us something about fundamental sociological concerns (with the operation of social systems, with the organization of work in society and with the enduring problems of power and control in social life), the study of behaviors which constitute those relations is profoundly important (cf. Waitzkin, 1979; 1983; and Waitzkin and Stoeckle, 1976). For example, how is scientific detachment conveyed in actual encounters between physicians and patients? How is the professional's stock of esoteric knowledge implemented in routine interactions with clients? Through what means is the licensed authority of a practitioner exercised in day-to-day communications with patients? And what is the relationship between other components of identity (such as race, class, or gender) and face-to-face engagements between doctors and their patients? Answers to questions such as these depend, in the first instance, on our systematic understanding of the organization of physician-patient interaction itself.

Approach and Overview of the Book

This is a book about actual encounters between doctors and patients in which I seek to treat talk between the two as a subject in its own right. Since my approach to the topic is closely linked to the origins of my interest in this area, a brief biographical sketch is perhaps in order here.

Recognition of the Problem

A few years ago, a national conference was held at a university campus to discuss "Women's Leadership and Authority in the Health Professions."[2] Invited participants represented a wide variety of fields (including nursing, pharmacology, sociology, psychology, social work, medicine, and women's studies). Among those invited were two women physicians.

For most who took part in the conference, it was an unqualified success. The papers were provocative, discussions spirited, and forums well-conceived. Judicious selection of contributors ensured that those in attendance were preeminent in their fields. Under these circumstances, it was hardly surprising to find the dialogue lively, and the overall experience of participation an exhilarating one.

Conveners of the conference organized a wine-and-cheese gathering on the last evening of the meeting. By that time, participants had a good deal to talk about, given previous illumination of their shared interests. However, as the party commenced, a sizable collection of people clustered around one of the two women physicians in attendance, creating a noticeable sociometric clumping in the room. The physician appeared to be holding forth on a topic of considerable interest, judging from the rapt expressions of those around her.

Drawing closer, I discovered that a question-and-answer session was actually in progress. Questions fired at the physician did not address her formal presentation at the meeting, even though that had been very well received. Nor did inquiries address her standing, as one of very few women who has "made it" in one of the best-paid and most sexually segregated professions in this country.[3] Instead, questions dealt with the everyday aches, pains, and ailments of the questioners themselves: "What can I do for recurrent cystitis?" asked one; "Can I really treat a yeast infection by douching with yogurt?" asked another; and "What do they mean by 'unspecified vaginitis?'" asked a third. Again and again, as the doctor offered her opinions, the questioners exclaimed: "My doctor never told me that!", "Nobody's ever explained this to me!", and "Why didn't he tell me!"

From the tones of both questions and answers, it was clear that this occasion constituted an earnest attempt to gain information, rather than merely solicitation of free medical advice. Remember that among those quizzing the physician were some of the best-established, most professionally acclaimed individuals in their fields. If people such as these were having trouble getting straight answers (or any answers at all) from their doctors, one might well wonder about the predicament of the average patient. These were educated, assertive professionals, with an intellectually active interest in health care—how much worse might the situation be for those less privileged?

The idea for this book, and for the five-year research project of which it is a part, was "born" at that conference. My previous research had suggested that power and control constitute significant aspects of many recurrent interactions, such as those between men and women and between parents and children. For example, in one earlier study, conducted with Don H. Zimmerman, I reported striking asymmetries in patterns of interruption in conversations between women and men recorded in natural settings: males initiated 96 percent of all interruptions which occurred there, and appeared to use interruptions to assert their rights to control topics of conversation (Zimmerman and West, 1975). Our later comparison of these conversations with a set of interactions between parents and children led us to suggest that females and children evidently receive similar treatment in conversations with males and with adults: both women and children are much more often interrupted by their conversational partners (West and Zimmerman, 1977). Even cross-sex conversations recorded in a laboratory setting between unacquainted college students displayed a much higher incidence of male-initiated than female-initiated interruption (West, 1979; 1982; West and Zimmerman, 1983). In short, these investigations indicated that the inequality between women and men exhibited in many macro-institutions in our society may have its parallel in at least part of one micro-institution. Of course, in our society, the doctor-patient relationship is frequently cited as the archetype of an unequal arrangement—where, it is supposed, one party has the power of "life and death" over the other.

Researching the Problem

People, however, rarely live up to their archetypal portrayals, and my own experiences over ten years of working as a pediatric medical assistant contradicted the popular stereotype of the all-powerful physician and all-helpless patient. Moreover, while reviewing the literature in medical journals in anticipation of beginning this research project, I repeatedly ran into articles dealing with the same "communication problems" that patients are wont to complain about, but written from the *physician's* point of view. Admittedly, many pieces in medical management periodicals tend to stress the part that misunderstandings play in reduced profits and efficiency. But the careful reader will find nearly as many essays bemoaning the costs of tangled lines of communication for more humanitarian reasons, including patients' health, welfare, and ongoing relationships with their doctors.

In concluding my overview of the medical literature, I reasoned that sociologists would have a great deal to say about these problems,

since theirs is the business of social relationships. Surprisingly, however, sociologists did not. The student of medical sociology or health
care will find an enormous amount of research addressed to structural and organizational features of medical practice, but compara-
tively little attention is paid to the micro-level concerns of day-to-day
interactions between physicians and their patients (for important exceptions, see Cicourel, 1981a; Fisher, 1983; Frankel, 1983; Heath,
1981; Mishler, 1984; Paget, 1983; Tannen and Wallat, 1983; and
Todd, 1983). As Chapter 2 will demonstrate, research in this area has
primarily been confined to abstract theory on the nature of the physician-patient relationship and a broad range of diverse empirical
studies that aim at increasing patient compliance, patient satisfaction,
and physician control in medical interviews. Seldom are studies found
that begin with what would seem to be the logical starting point for
investigations of physician-patient communication—namely, a systematic description of talk between doctors and patients.

One obvious impediment to such research is, of course, the confidentiality of the physician-patient relationship. Given that what goes
on between doctors and patients is generally regarded as privileged
information, it is understandable that social scientists might encounter problems gaining access to actual exchanges between the two.
Thus, many suggestions on improving communication between doctors and patients come from research which employs questionnaires.
Although such research yields many helpful insights into physicians'
and patients' attitudes, the questionnaire format is not equipped to
say much about their behaviors. While a few studies have dealt with
the exchange of talk between doctors and patients, they typically lack
any explicit model of speech exchange in terms of which their findings can be interpreted.

An appropriate model can be found, however, in conversation analysis, which provides a systematic approach to the study of talk as a
topic in its own right. Conversation analysis is concerned with the
social organization of conversational interaction.[4] Within this framework, regularly occurring features of interaction are seen as methodical solutions to situated technical problems that interactants must
"solve." For example, Sacks (1966) has observed that children frequently use the form "D'ya know what?" when initiating talk with
adults. Rather than eliminating this observation as extraneous or in-
cidental to "real" conversational topics, Sacks analyzed its routine oc-

currence as a result of children's special problems in gaining adults' attention and engaging them in conversation. The answer to "D'ya know what?" is ordinarily another question of the form "What?" and the adult so responding finds that he or she has given the child opportunity to speak and be listened to—at least for the moment. In this example, "D'ya know what?" is viewed as a methodical solution to problems associated with children's restricted rights to speak. More generally, this approach to interactional data allows us to examine the procedures speakers use to open up, sustain, and shut down a state of talk in terms of the interactional "work" that they do (see Frankel and Beckman, 1981, for an application of this approach to the opening of medical encounters). Subsequent chapters of this book employ conversation analysis to address the social organization of medical dialogues as a topic in and of itself.

Admittedly, the topic is a vast one. A decisive body of work on the organization of physician-patient interaction might encompass many volumes. Since this book constitutes an exploratory investigation, there are many avenues of study it will leave untouched. For example, such important channels of nonverbal communication as eye contact, facial expression, and body orientation must also be given systematic attention in order to provide a complete description of the structure of interaction between doctors and patients. Moreover, the analyses of verbal exchange presented here will suggest many further areas of investigation on the organization of talk itself. Thus, this book should be read as a preliminary exploration of a much neglected area of research, rather than as the final word on the subject.

But while my selection of analytic foci is an arbitrary one, it is far from capricious. The problems addressed here (turn-taking between physicians and patients; the organization of questions and answers, repairs of misunderstandings, and sociable commentary in medical discourse) represent some of the major organizational issues confronting analysts of face-to-face interaction:

> In any society, whenever the physical possibility of spoken interaction arises, it seems that a system of practices, conventions, and procedural rules comes into play which functions as a means of guiding and organizing the flow of messages. An understanding will prevail as to when and where it will be permissible to initiate talk, among whom, and by means of what topic of conversation. A set of significant gestures is employed to initiate a spate of communication and as a means for the

persons concerned to accredit each other as legitimate participants. (Goffman, 1967:33–34)

Goffman's description highlights the fundamental nature of the sorts of concerns represented in this volume: By what means is an orderly exchange of turns at talk effected in medical discourse? How do physicians and patients employ questions and answers to exchange information with one another? What are their resources for managing ambiguities and misunderstandings between themselves? And, what parts do aspects of sociable chitchat play in the construction of social relations between doctor and patient? These are some of the substantive problems the work addresses.

The Data

The data for this book consist primarily of 532 pages of transcribed two-party encounters between physicians and patients recorded in a family practice center in the southern United States. Chapter 3 is addressed to the "how" and "why" of this particular data collection.

Physicians in these encounters were residents in a family practice residency program, which requires three years of additional training beyond medical school. Thus, the physicians are typically young (early to mid-thirties) when in training at the Center. The encounters I analyze include fourteen male physicians and four female physicians[5]; all eighteen are white.

Patients in these interactions range in age from sixteen to eighty-two years: 4 were in their teens; 9 were under forty; and 7 were over fifty at the time of recording. The patients include 5 white males, 4 black males, 6 white females and 5 black females. In socioeconomic status, the 20 patients evidenced a variety of backgrounds, including that of professional worker, housewife, construction worker, unemployed carpenter, and domestic worker.

The encounters I analyze were actual "visits to the doctor," and thus are not standardized for duration of interaction, purpose of visit, or length of relationship between physician and patient. Clearly, there are costs and benefits attached to the analysis of such a corpus of materials (see Chapter 3). This collection of medical exchanges does not, of course, constitute a random sample of conversationalists or conversations. So, simple projections from findings based on this collection to doctors, patients, or medical dialogues at large cannot be justified by the usual logic of statistical inference. The stability of any empirical finding cannot, in any event, be established by a single study.

What, then, can be learned from such a diverse assembly of patients, specialized subsegment of physicians, and sample of this size? The first advantage offered by a study of this nature is a detailed description of the ways in which physicians and patients *do* interact with one another in their natural setting. The family practice center at which they were recorded has employed audiotaping and videotaping for several years as a part of the medical training of residents. With patients' signed consent, they are recorded with their doctors by means of ceiling microphones and unobtrusive cameras located in the corners of examination rooms. After recordings are made, faculty at the Center review tapes with the residents, and provide suggestions for improving treatment and diagnostic procedures. Hence, the tapes were not produced for purposes of my research, but were subsequently transcribed for these purposes. They are thus an "unmotivated" source for study, in keeping with standards of conversation analysis. Transcribing the tapes entailed a ten-week stay at the medical setting, where I got to know many of the medical faculty and residents fairly well. My relationships with them provide anecdotal material throughout the book, which—while not part of the data base proper—adds an additional source of subjective interpretation by the physicians themselves.

The second major contribution offered by an investigation of this sort is illustration of a new method of investigating the physician-patient relationship. As noted earlier, existing theoretical formulations of this relationship provide no clear direction for assessing their empirical adequacy. Moreover, many inconsistencies in empirical research result from methodological discrepancies arising through lack of coherent theoretical bases for interpretation of results. Conversation analysis proposes that the linkage of particular classes of verbal behaviors with particular social activities cannot be derived by application of an analyst's pre-specified categorizations; rather, it must be extracted from the conversational practices of speakers themselves by approaching the study of talk as an activity or topic in its own right.

Were this a study of physicians' or patients' characteristics, the data I have collected would be ill-suited for generalizing beyond the physicians and patients here described. The physicians are, after all, family practice residents. Thus, they are typically just beginning medical practice in one of the most progressive specialties in modern medicine.[6] The patients, further, cannot be said to constitute a representative sample of all persons who consult physicians. Pediatric interviews are, by deliberate intent, excluded from consideration (see Chapter 3), and emergency visits are generally conducted at a nearby hospital rather than on the premises of the family practice center.

However, there is within these data a set of locally occurring technical problems that physicians and patients must solve in the course of their talk together. My argument rests on the assumption that these problems (e.g., opening up a state of talk, sustaining an ongoing interaction through verbal and nonverbal practices, and terminating an exchange) are not idiosyncratic problems faced by these particular physicians and patients at this particular time. Rather, they are technical problems which must be faced *whenever* physicians and patients come together for purposes of conducting an exchange.[7] So, regardless of the identities of the particular physicians and patients in this collection of medical interviews, I believe that the stability and orderliness of their interactional patterns are products of locally occasioned (but trans-situational) problems posed by the interaction itself.

The third promise of this study rests in its potential use as grounding and as a point of departure for further investigations. The book will not serve as an alternative "Guide to Understanding Your Doctor," nor is it intended to do so. Rather, its primary contribution lies in its empirical analysis of how understanding and misunderstanding occur in the first instance. The study can be used to assess sociological formulations of the patient-practitioner relationship within the concrete, day-to-day situations in which it is constructed. Further, it promises the student of face-to-face interaction a grounded methodology for exploring the dynamics of micropolitical encounters.

Organization Of The Book

This first chapter was intended to introduce the reader to the general problems associated with physician-patient interaction. Chapter 2 presents an overview of existing research on the doctor-patient relationship and physician-patient communication. In Chapter 3, I provide a discussion of the approach of conversation analysis and the collection of physicians, patients, and medical exchanges analyzed in this book. For purposes of convenience and internal cohesion, I have organized the remaining chapters around the sorts of regularly occurring problems physicians and patients encounter when conducting conversations with one another. In these four chapters (4, 5, 6, and 7), findings of my research are presented on the organization of turns at talk (Chapter 4), the exchange of questions and answers (Chapter 5), the resolution of misunderstandings (Chapter 6) and the initiation of laughter and social commentary (Chapter 7) between physicians and patients.[8] The final chapter (Chapter 8) offers a reconsideration of doctor-patient discourse as a social organizational issue and the summary and conclusions of this research.

CHAPTER 2

The Study of Doctor-Patient Communication

"Communication" is not listed in the index to many social science texts on health care. Somewhere between "communicable diseases" and "community health centers" the topic is altogether lost. Nevertheless, the perseverant reader will find information pertinent to this subject under the general rubric of "the physician-patient relationship." Wilson's (1970) explanation does much to account for this particular mode of indexing:

> Patient-practitioner relationships are best viewed in the framework of social roles, of the attitudes and activities the two parties bring to the situation of care. This interaction of two or more persons, centering around the health needs of a single individual, is far from being a spontaneous happening. It is, rather, a more or less well-rehearsed confrontation in which the key participants have learned to expect certain things and to act in certain ways. (p. 14)

If, as Wilson contends, the "script" is already written for physicians and patients, the neglect of communication as a topic within the sociology of health is understandable. From the analyst's view, the only problematic aspect of doctor-patient interaction concerns participants' appropriate assumption of the social roles of physician and patient.

To understand how this perspective evolved and how instrumental a part it has played in tracking social scientific ideas on the subject, it is necessary to go back to the theoretical framework of the physician-patient relationship initially formulated by Parsons in 1951.

The Doctor-Patient Relationship

Parsons's (1951) original analytic interest in health care was in medical practice as a subsystem of the larger structure of social action in Western society. Given his focus on the organization of social systems, he approached the physician-patient relationship as an institutionalized role set, consisting of standardized behavioral expectations for patient and practitioner.

Those standardized behavioral expectations were seen to revolve around the patient's need for help from the physician. As Parsons put it: "The patient has a need for technical services because he doesn't—nor do his lay associates, family members, etc.—'know' what is the matter or what to do about it, nor does he control the necessary facilities. The physician is the technical expert who by special training and experience, and by an institutionally validated status, is qualified to "help" the patient in a situation institutionally defined as legitimate in a relative sense but as needing help" (1951:439). "Help," in this paradigm, means restoration to a nonpathological state. Central to the framework is the idea that illness can be seen as a form of deviance; that is, a form of disturbance of the healthy functioning of the total organism within the social system. Institutionalization of the patient-practitioner relationship is thus warranted to ensure maintenance of society (to which illness poses a major threat).

An Asymmetrical Relationship

Because it is the physician, within Western cultures, who is charged with the legal responsibility for restoring the patient to normality, "The practitioner must have control over the interaction with the patient, ensuring that the patient will comply with the prescribed regimen. If patient compliance is not ensured, then the ability of the practitioner to return the patient to a normal functioning state is undermined" (Wolinsky, 1980:163). The essential *asymmetry* of the physician-patient relationship is, for Parsons, the key to the therapeutic practice of medicine. He equates the practitioner's interactional control over patients with the ability to treat them.

Physicians' control or power over patients derives from three sources. First, patients are in a position of situational dependency vis-à-vis their doctors, in that they recognize their need for health care and their inability to provide it for themselves. Second, physicians are in a position of situational authority vis-à-vis patients, since only doctors possess the specialized knowledge and technical qualifications required to provide medical services. Third, physicians' professional prestige provides them an additional edge in their interactions with patients. The technical skills they acquire through medical training and their societal certification as licensed healers afford physicians what Wolinsky describes as "a nonpareil social position in modern society. Therefore, in almost any social situation, the practitioner commands more respect and more prestige than does the patient. As a result, in everyday and *especially* health related interaction, the practitioner commands and receives deference from others, allowing the practitioner to dominate interpersonal encounters" (1980:164). Within the Parsonian framework, then, the doctor-patient relationship is *predicated* on institutionalized inequality between those who heal and those who must come to them for treatment.

MODIFICATIONS OF THE MODEL

Originally formulated in 1951, expanded in 1952 (Parsons and Fox), and reiterated in 1975, Parsons's model of the physician-patient relationship remains the classic approach to social interaction between doctors and patients. Nonetheless, critics of this model have been many (see Bloom and Wilson, 1979, and Wolinsky, 1980:166–185, for excellent overviews of these).

Illness and the Sick Role

Some have suggested that Parsons neglected the roles of other actors in the health-care process (such as members of the patient's family, or the ever-increasing staff of personnel involved in medical services). The physician-patient relationship, notes Bloom (1963), is only one component in a larger sociocultural matrix of health care consumers and providers.

Freidson (1961; 1970a; 1970b; 1975) goes even further, avowing that patients' lay associates in fact comprise a distinct referral system, with dynamics of its own. For example: "What medicine comes to define as an illness is in part a function of the way its experience is limited by the characteristics of the laymen who happen to enter the consulting room. . . . Not a representative sample of the population. . . . The grounds for selection are not the profession's conceptions of

illness, and the organization of the process is in important ways independent of the organization of the profession" (Freidson, 1970b:279).
Thus, Freidson maintains that the relationship between doctor and
patient cannot be fully understood without analyzing lay construc-⌉
tions of illness, independently of practitioners' definitions of it.   ⌋

Considerable research supports the view that patients' "pathways to
the doctor" are rife with ambiguity and conflicting perspectives (Zola,
1973). For example, cultural differences between patients figure cen-
trally in differing attitudes toward physical symptoms and differential
responses to pain (Zborowski, 1958; Croog, 1961; Zola, 1963; 1966;
Stoeckle et al., 1963; 1964; Becker, 1979). Varying interpretations of
the meaning of symptoms are also found among patients of different
ages, sexes, levels of education, and socioeconomic statuses (Feldman,
1966; Hetherington and Hopkins, 1969; Banks and Keller, 1971;
Guttmacher and Elinson, 1971; and Mechanic, 1972). A review of
these findings leads Becker (1979) to conclude: "Perhaps Parsons'
(1951:436) original formulation of the [patient's] 'sick role' is meaningful only in terms of particular sociocultural influences on the role's
behavioral expectations" (p. 261).

The Role of the Physician

Parsons's (1951) characterization of the physician's role has also
stimulated considerable controversy, particularly among researchers
with interests in medicine as a profession. For example, Freidson
(1970b) questions the extent to which values comprising the physician's presumed "collectivity orientation" (achievement, universalism,
functional specificity, and affective neutrality) are evidenced in clinical practice: "Parsons does not specify performance at all, but broad
institutional norms connected with professions as officially organized
occupations. . . . They are quite distinct, analytically and empirically,
from the actual norms of individual professionals" (p. 160). In practice, Freidson observes, the norms and attitudes governing medical
work foster a personal and restricted sense of responsibility. Drawing
on the classic investigation of students at the University of Kansas
Medical School by Becker et al. (1961), Freidson argues that the organization of medical work necessitates a particularistic (rather than
collectivistic) orientation to action and concrete experience. Physicians' particularistic orientation can be seen not only in the ways they
handle professional self-regulation (in matters of unethical or incom-

petent behavior), but also in their dealings with patients. Hence, Freidson contends that medical sociology should address itself to the ways in which medical work is organized in health-care settings rather than to characteristics of health care personnel (e.g., their training, sensitivity, or devotion).

Although Freidson (1961; 1970a; 1970b; 1975) is credited with the most comprehensive challenge to Parsons (Anderson and Helm, 1979:260; Bloom and Wilson, 1979:285–288), others have made substantial contributions to a new approach (e.g., Becker et al., 1961; Bucher and Stelling, 1969; Davis, 1964; Hughes, 1971; Roth, 1963b; Strauss, 1970; Glaser and Strauss, 1965; Scheff, 1963). Underlying all these works are a perspective emphasizing the clash of perspectives between doctor and patient, and the three basic premises of symbolic interactionism:

1. Human beings act toward things on the basis of the meanings that things have for them.
2. Meaning derives from social interaction.
3. Meanings are modified by their interpretations, used by persons in actual situations. (Blumer, 1969:2)

Within this theoretical framework, such matters as health and illness are seen as the products of negotiated interactions between health-care consumers and providers (see Anderson and Helm, 1979, for a helpful overview of this approach). Thus, the empirical studies derived from this view have focused on the social construction of meanings in medical contexts (e.g., Ball, 1967; Becker et al., 1961; Conrad and Kern, 1981; Daniels, 1973; Danziger, 1980; 1981; Emerson, 1970; Freidson, 1961).

Such studies frequently employ particular instances of language use to illuminate the ways in which medical realities are created and sustained. For example, Danziger's (1980) analysis of physicians' terminology in obstetric visits displayed the channeling of "possible prenatals" into bona fide pregnant women. Despite suggestive clinical evidence (e.g., positive pregnancy tests), doctors in her study were loathe to categorize women as "prenatals" until their full medical workups were completed. Emerson's (1970) investigation of gynecological encounters found medical providers using definite articles rather than pronoun adjectives when alluding to patients' body parts. Directives with sexual connotations were shunned, and euphemistic references substituted for them wherever possible (see chapter 3 for further discussion).

However, here, as in Parsons's (1951) formulations, talk between physicians and patients is utilized as a resource rather than as an object of investigation: Meanings *derive* from social interaction, but meanings themselves are the proper subjects of study. Hence, works such as Emerson's (1970) invoke various aspects of medical talk in explaining how medical realities are sustained (pp. 80–85), but the principles organizing talk itself remain unaddressed (see Frankel, 1983:25, n. 9).

The Need for Asymmetry in Therapeutic Relations

Other critics have questioned the characterization of patients' passivity implied by Parsons's (1951) discussion of their situational dependency.[1] For example, Szasz and Hollender (1956) contend that the severity of physiological symptoms is likely to influence the extent to which patients are dependent on their doctors. Thus, the traumatized, comatose, or otherwise unconscious patient is literally helpless to participate in his or her own care; under these circumstances it would of course be nonsensical to speak of a patient's "active" role in the health-care process. However, less extreme symptoms (such as those which are likely to accompany mumps or flu) are unlikely to totally incapacitate patients. So, Szasz and Hollender argue, patients seeking medical treatment for less incapacitating problems are perfectly capable of playing a larger role in their own health care; they may be looking for guidance from and cooperating with physicians, rather than being totally dominated by them. Finally, they contend that ongoing treatment of chronic but nonincapacitating conditions (e.g., allergies or diabetes mellitus) requires *mutual* participation by patients and physicians. Under these circumstances, patients usually carry out prescribed regimens (such as insulin injections) themselves with periodic visits to their physicians (see also Danziger, 1981, on pregnancy care).

Wolinsky (1980) adds an important point to Szasz and Hollender's typology of patient responsibility, noting that the "mutual participation" model also seems applicable to cases in which preventive medicine is the issue. Routine physical examinations, for example, are likely to involve patients as well as doctors in the development and implementation of strategies for continued good health. However,

Wolinsky warns that this pseudo-egalitarian form of the physician-patient relationship requires considerable sophistication on the part of patients, "limiting the applicability of the mode to mature, informed adults. As such, the mutual participation model of the patient-practitioner relationship is analogous to the relationship of one adult to another with one adult having the specialized knowledge needed by the other" (1980:174). In summary, Wolinsky contends that Szasz and Hollender's modifications amount to a "recalibration" of the Parsonian model—subdividing the child-parent character of the original into "infant-parent, adolescent-parent, and adult-adult" life stages (p. 174). We are left then, with a relationship between physician and patient which is still fundamentally asymmetrical.

In fact, Parsons's response to his critics (1975) re-emphasizes the *necessity* for institutionalized asymmetry in physicians' relationships with patients. While it is true, he acknowledges, that instances of self-treatment and successful folk remedies can be found, "these marginal cases . . . cannot legitimately be used as a model for the institutionalization of these types of functions" (p. 277). To illustrate this point, Parsons draws an analogy between the physician-patient relationship and the professor-student relationship. In the latter, he contends, teachers are in the position of certified social control agents who are allocated the legal responsibility for eradicating ignorance and incompetence. Students may, of course, learn some things on their own; they may be self-taught in particular matters. Nonetheless, it is the professor rather than the student who is entrusted with the responsibility for imparting and evaluating the knowledge and competence required of cultural members. The societal certification of this responsibility (e.g., through professors' academic credentials and training, through accreditation procedures for institutions of higher learning, and through prerequisites of certain educational degrees for particular jobs) institutionalizes the essential asymmetry of the professor-student relationship. As in the case of practitioner-patient relations, the therapeutic character of the interaction requires an asymmetrical distribution of power and authority if, as Wolinsky quips, the ignorant are to be "healed" (p. 172).

In contrast to this situation, Parsons (1975) notes three types of social relationships which are predicated on an equal distribution of power. The first is that of a free market system, in which, he argues, continued participation is contingent on continued economic interest.

The second is that of a voluntary or democratic organization, in which, he suggests, all members are officially declared to be equals even though elected leadership positions may rotate among members. The third and most interesting example Parsons chooses to character-ize symmetrical social relationships is that of a communications network.

By "communication," Parsons—like many other organizational the-orists—means an exchange of information. Here, parties to commu-nication processes are assumed to have equal access to the symbolic meaning of information they transmit in order to communicate at all.

Herein lies a curious paradox. If, as Parsons argues, communica-tion is predicated on *symmetrical* relations, and if, as he also contends, the practitioner-patient relationship is *essentially* asymmetrical, then communication between physicians and patients is theoretically im-possible. Exchange is prohibited when parties to communication processes do not have equal access to the symbolic meaning of infor-mation they transmit.

More to the point, for present purposes, is the fact that Parsons (1951; Parsons and Fox, 1952; Parsons, 1975) provides a theoretical formulation of the relationship between physicians and patients, rather than an empirical investigation of their interactions with one another. My argument is not that theory and empirical work are incompatible, but that any formulation of the relationship between doctors and patients ought to be grounded in the empirical analysis of interactions between them. To find such empirical research, the reader must consult a very different and diverse set of sources.

COMPLIANCE, SATISFACTION, AND CONTROL

Noticeably absent in traditional sociological discussions of the doc-tor-patient relationship, empirical studies of medical dialogues are nonetheless abundant in a diverse body of research on patient com-pliance, patient satisfaction, and physician control (see Pendleton, 1983; Stone, 1979, and Waitzkin, 1983, for excellent reviews of this work).[2] Korsch and Negrete's (1972) now classic study puts forth the rationale for these investigations most convincingly: "The quality of medical care depends in the last analysis on the interaction of the patient and the doctor, and there is abundant evidence that in current practice this interaction all too often is disappointing to both parties"

(p. 66). Korsch and Negrete find considerable reason for patients' disappointment in their doctors. In more than half of the 800 visits they investigated, physicians resorted to arcane medical terminology which mystified their patients; in less than 5 percent of cases was the physician's conversation of a friendly or sociable sort; and in fully 26 percent of instances, the chief worries of those initiating the visit were never mentioned, since physicians provided them no opportunities to do so.

Such findings might lead one to conclude that "solutions" to problems of physician-patient communication are relatively straightforward: (1) eliminate medical jargon, (2) cultivate sociable conversation between physicians and patients, and (3) expand the length of sessions to permit patients' expression of their chief concerns. Would that it were so simple.

Conceptual Problems

Although medical "jargon" is a recurring theme in empirical studies, research on its effects yields findings which are often contradictory. Korsch and Negrete, for example, imply that doctors tend to talk over their patients' heads—certainly ample reason for patients' confusion. McKinlay (1975), however, finds that doctors consistently *underestimate* patients' knowledge of medical terms—which would suggest that physicians tend to talk "down" to their patients.[3] To complicate matters further, Wallen et al. (1979) report that (male) physicians are more likely to err in estimates of their patients' knowledge when the patients are female; with women patients, physicians underestimate *and* overestimate more frequently than with patients who are men. Other studies (e.g., Pendleton and Bochner, 1980; Hayes-Bautista, 1978) report variations in the successful transmission of medical information by patients' ethnicity and social class. In short, it seems that patients do not like medical jargon, but physicians do not know what constitutes it.[4]

The significance of longer time to satisfaction with medical dialogues is also unclear (e.g., Bain, 1979; Brody and Stokes, 1970; Parrish et al., 1967). Korsch and Negrete hypothesized that time would be positively correlated with patient satisfaction, that is, patients would be more satisfied when physicians spent more time interacting with them. Yet they found no significant relationship between the two factors. Neither patient satisfaction nor clarity of doctors' diagnoses improved when sessions took longer. In fact, longer exchanges often were a product of interactional problems, where patients and physicians spent time trying to resolve communication failures. Another study (Cartwright et al., 1974) found physicians tend to be less satisfied when interviews consume more of their time, particularly when longer exchanges were a function of patients talking more. Commonsense cannot quite explain away these results: In tacit agreement with the old maxim which states "Time is money," physicians' fee schedules provide for charging more for longer patient visits (e.g., initial office visits, complete physicals or referrals). Hence, the rationale for physician dissatisfaction with longer interviews is not immediately obvious.

However, some light is shed on this subject by coupling Korsch and Negrete's findings with the results obtained by Wallen et al. In the latter investigation, the authors note that male physicians offer more explanations to their female patients than their male patients. But male physicians spend no more *time* in so doing. In other words, "the men may have received fewer but fuller explanations than the women" in the same amount of time (1979:145). Perfunctory explanations could certainly account for both patients' and physicians' dissatisfaction with longer exchanges. Here, as in the case of parents who are employed outside the home, it may be that the quantity of time is not as important as the quality of time spent in interaction. Unfortunately, Wallen and her associates only transcribed the "information-exchange" portions of interviews they recorded, so their findings do not encompass those portions of exchanges that may have been spent in "miscellaneous, or social, comments" (1979:139).

"Social comments" and sociable conversation often have been categorized as extraneous or inappropriate to the structure of physician-patient interactions. A host of studies (Berkowitz et al., 1963; Davis, 1968; Elling et al., 1960; Ley and Spelman, 1965) relate patients' compliance with medical advice to malfunctions in the communication process. Malfunctions, it seems, may result from sociable remarks that obscure the underlying asymmetry of the physician-patient relationship. Davis (1968), for example, finds that noncompliance occurs more often when patients give their own opinions and when physicians display "permissive acceptance" of patients' active participation. He concludes that passive patients are more likely to comply with medical advice. As he explains:

Presumably, all doctors and patients have certain ideas about the kind of relationships they *should* have, and the kind of roles they are expected to play. . . . Implicit in this discussion of noncompliance is the problem of controlling patient behavior. In the doctor-patient relationship, whether in private practice, hospital clinic, or on a ward, the doctor must rely on his ability to establish good rapport in order to inculcate in his patient a positive orientation and commitment to their relationship so that ultimately the patient will follow his advice. (Davis, 1968:284)

Like Parsons, Davis appears to equate interactional control over patients with the ability to treat them: a "good" rapport is one in which the physician's control over the patient is clearly evidenced. Leventhal (1965) carries this one step further, suggesting that the arousal of fear in patients is necessary in order to ensure their compliance with doctors' orders.

Korsch and Negrete contradict these suggestions, finding that physician "friendliness" contributes positively to patient satisfaction. In their study, which actually treated parents as patients in pediatric interviews, the "active" parent was more likely to comply than the "passive" one, and the permissiveness of the physician made no difference at all. Since Korsch and Negrete also stress the importance of good rapport between doctor and patient, they could be seen as concluding that good communication does *not* depend on the archetypal relationship thought to exist between omnipotent physicians and "helpless" patients. Of what, then, does good communication consist?

Methodological Issues

Contradictions between Davis (1968) and Korsch and Negrete (1972) provide a good focal point for discussing the methodological problems that have plagued researchers in this area. One set of difficulties has arisen with the use of elicited responses (in interviews and questionnaires) in analyses of doctor-patient communication. Such researchers as Collins (1955), Skipper (1965), and McKinlay (1975) have relied on this technique, and in so doing have limited the scope of their findings to physicians' and patients' reconstructed *perceptions* of the communication between them. While it is important to know what patients think of their doctors' verbal behaviors (and vice versa), it is also important to distinguish these perceptions from the behaviors themselves. For example, McKinlay (as noted above) discovered that physicians *thought* patients knew less medical terminology than they actually did. Despite my earlier suggestions, this does not necessarily mean that doctors talk down to their patients. In fact, McKinlay finds that physicians express willingness to use technical language *even though* they think their patients will not understand it. However, as Frankel (forthcoming) notes, whether or not physicians deliberately intend to deceive, obscure, or limit the flow of information to patients, "How the patient actually behaves or receives dominating or limiting communication from the physician, and of course, physician's subsequent response is left unaddressed as a topic or focus for research" (p. 26: fn. 8). The questionnaire format, used in written or oral form, simply is not designed to investigate these issues.

Seeking to sidestep such difficulties, some studies (Davis, 1968; Svarstad and Lipton, 1977) have used content analyses of tapes and medical records to achieve a more objective measure of doctors' and patients' behaviors. Svarstad and Lipton, for example, employed an innovative index of physicians' "frankness" when discussing mental retardation with the parents of mentally retarded children. Part of the study's design included a comparison of clinicians' actual words (which had been recorded on audiotape as the interview progressed) with their responses to a post-interview questionnaire. The questionnaire asked physicians for their diagnostic categorization of childrens' handicaps (e.g., "mildly retarded," "moderately retarded"); the content analysis assessed the extent to which this was actually communicated to parents (e.g., as "a bit slow," "behind others of this age"). If physicians' words to parents were identical to those they used in their questionnaire responses, their communications were defined as "frank." If, on the other hand, they used words that were different, particularly in ways which might lead parents to alternative estimations of the childrens' handicaps, their communications were defined as "vague." The researchers found a significant relationship between physicians' frankness and subsequent parental "acceptance" of childrens' retardation.

However, they note that candid and specific information does not *ensure* acceptance by parents:

> We suspect that it would be fruitful to analyze how the parents' attitudes are affected when the professional provides additional information and/ or other types of communication . . . is there a point at which the professional provides so much detail that it leads to parental confusion, hopelessness and rejection? Do certain amounts and types of supportive

communication (e.g. reassurance, encouragement) increase parental acceptance of the child's handicap? . . . "Frankness" means different things
to different people. (Svarstad and Lipton, 1977:650–651)

To these insightful points, I would add a further concern: How are
physicians to "know," in the context of actual interviews, what parents
are thinking? In this study, of course, researchers gained access to
parents' perceptions in a post-visit research interview. But in everyday
life, physicians have no way of assessing parental (or patient) reactions
to words that they use *as they use them* other than by observing parents'
responses then and there. This would suggest an alternative methodology to those measures Svarstad and Lipton employed; namely,
the analysis of the interaction *between* physicians and patients as it
actually occurs.

It was to achieve this end that Bales (1950) devised Interaction
Process Analysis. Used for some time to study leadership and authority in experimental small groups, this methodology has also been
employed to assess satisfaction, compliance, and control in physician-
patient exchanges (Davis, 1968; Korsch and Negrete, 1972; see also
Lennard and Bernstein, 1960; and Gottschalk and Gleser, 1969, for
its use in the analysis of therapist-client interactions). Interaction
Process Analysis has made a major contribution to the study of
doctor-patient communication by providing a means of examining
interactional developments over time rather than limiting analysis to
the outcomes of those developments (e.g., what was "finally" understood, or who had "the last word" in making a medical decision).
However, the evidence provided by Bales's system is inconclusive,
and, at times, contradictory.

For example, I introduced this discussion of methodological issues
by noting discrepancies between Davis's (1968) and Korsch and Negrete's (1972) conclusions on patient compliance: Davis suggested
that passive patients were more likely to comply, while Korsch and
Negrete argued that active patients were more likely to do so. The
disagreement of these researchers is all the more striking in light of
the fact that both employed the same method, Interaction Process
Analysis, to obtain their results. It is possible, of course, that selection
of different samples might have contributed to different findings:
Davis examined interactions between physicians and patients in a general medical clinic, while Korsch and Negrete looked at exchanges
between pediatricians and mothers at a large teaching hospital.

But Svarstad (1979) argues that the likely problem with both sets of findings is the Bales system itself. The categories it uses are too broad, she contends:

> For example, the extent to which the physician gives instruction or suggestion can be measured, but the content, clarity, or salience of the suggestions or instructions cannot be explored. The extent to which the physician expresses positive or negative affect can be measured, but the other ways in which the physician might try to motivate the patient (e.g., discussing the rationale for a given prescription) cannot be isolated. The latter communication would be included in broad categories such as "giving orientation" or "giving opinions." (p. 248)

I would suggest that narrowing the breadth of Bales's categories would not, by itself, solve all the problems associated with this mode of analysis. As Simon and Boyer (1968:1) note, interaction analysis systems are explicitly interested in that which "can be categorized or measured." Typically, categorization consists of coding ongoing interaction into pre-specified classifications, which, in turn, are organized and interpreted on the basis of the analyst's typifications (e.g., as "active" versus "passive" behaviors). Delamont and Hamilton (1976:8) argue that these systems may utilize "crude measurement techniques which are characterized by ill-defined boundaries between the categories (e.g., the distinction between "acceptance" and "encouragement" of another's opinion). Still other critics question the applicability of interaction process analysis to interactions occurring outside the context of task-oriented experimental small groups (cf. Bernard, 1972; Laws, 1971; and Slater, 1961). In other words, while interaction analysis systems may be, as some have claimed (e.g., Flanders, 1970), highly *reliable* methods of measurement, their validity is not beyond question (see Mishler, 1979, especially pp. 6–7). In fact, as Delamont and Hamilton (1976:9) propose, they "may assume the truth of what they claim to be explaining."

To reiterate, conventional empirical studies of physician-patient interaction have suffered from three major methodological problems. First the use of questionnaires is sufficient for investigations of doctors' and patients' perceptions of communication, but not for assessments of their actual behavior. Second, the use of content analysis tends to abstract the "what" and "how much" of speech events from the "when," "where" and "why" of their occurrence. And third, the use of Interaction Process Analysis further compounds this problem by raising initially ambiguous measurement procedures to an even higher level of abstraction.

DISCOURSE ANALYSIS

Since about 1975, the study of interaction between doctors and patients has been transfused by new blood from a variety of donors (e.g., Cicourel, 1975; 1977; 1981a; 1982; Gumperz, 1982; Hymes, 1974; Labov and Fanshel, 1977; Mishler, 1979; in press). Traditional academic disciplines are well represented here by sociology, anthropology, linguistics, and psychology. More important, however, are the various approaches to discourse that have emerged within these fields: for example, ethnographies of communication (Hymes, 1974; Phillips, 1977), speech act analyses and expansions thereof (Labov and Fanshel, 1977; Gumperz, 1982; Tannen, in press; Tannen and Wallat, 1983), phenomenologies of talk (Mishler, in press; Paget, 1983), and cognitive sociologies of discourse (Cicourel, 1978; 1980a; 1981b; 1983; Fisher, 1983; Fisher and Todd, 1983a; Måseide, 1983; Todd, 1983). While works in these genres share no single tradition (cf. Cicourel, 1980b; Gumperz, 1982:153–171; Labov and Fanshel, 1977:19–28, Mishler, 1984: Chapter 2), all are tied to one another—and to the purposes of this book—by an important common denominator: "They examine meticulously at least some details of recorded verbal behavior" (Labov and Fanshel, 1977:19). In this respect, discourse analyses differ dramatically from other empirical studies of physician-patient communication (cf. Pendleton, 1983). Conventional concerns with outcome variables (e.g., satisfaction and compliance) are suspended in the interests of substantiating relationships between discourse and context (see Fisher and Todd, 1983b: 1–17).

However, despite a shared emphasis on the social production of talk in situated contexts, discourse analysis differs in epistemology from conversation analysis—the approach utilized in this book (see Chapter 3). In part, the distinction between the two centers on the differential roles of meaning attributed to speakers' productions. Whereas conversation analysis is concerned with the systematic organization of talk as a topic unto itself, discourse analysis is prompted by a further motivation:

It explores the consequences of . . . differences in beliefs and expectations for a medical interview and examination, yielding an explication of how communication works and does not work *and how meaning gets encoded in and decoded from talk in medical settings.* (Tannen and Wallet, 1983:203; emphasis added)

The researcher seeks to create *a causal network which will account for the content of the discourse or text.* We identify the persons involved, their perceptions, their goals, their intentions, their actions, their evaluation of the events and settings, and the consequences of what was tried and not done or avoided. (Cicourel, 1980b:121; emphasis added)

Two questions are relevant in the analysis (1) *What is meant by the exchange? What does it reflect about the speaker's state of mind* and his relationship to the [other]? (2) By what verbal devices are the relevant effects obtained? Are there any special features of style, pronunciation or vocabulary which are significant? (Gumperz, 1972: 222; emphasis added)

But the fundamental schism between discourse analysis and conversation analysis derives from a deeper divergence. As Schegloff observes:

The common discourse-analytic standpoint treats the lecture, or sermon, or story told in an elicitation interview, campfire setting, or around the table, as the product of a single speaker and a single mind; the conversation-analytic angle of inquiry will not let go of the fact that speech-exchange systems are involved, in which more than one participant is present and relevant to the talk, even when only one does any talking. (1981:1–2)

Thus, just as discourse analysts suspend conventional concerns (with such outcome variables as satisfaction and compliance) in their studies of physician-patient interaction, conversation analysts suspend discourse-analytic concerns (with beliefs, intentions, and "states of mind" of individual participants) while attending to the detailed organization of talk itself.

SUMMARY AND CONCLUSIONS

Despite widespread concern over problems associated with doctor-patient communication, social science has offered few guidelines for potential solutions. As we have seen, research in this area has been confined primarily to abstract theory on the nature of the physician-patient relationship and a diverse set of empirical studies focused on

patient compliance, patient satisfaction, and physician control (excepted from this generalization are the discourse analyses reviewed
just above).

Theoretical work is largely indebted to Parsons's framework, which
stressed the extent to which the physician-patient relationship consists
of institutionalized behavioral expectations, such as the affective neutrality of the physician's role or the situational dependency of the
patient's. While subsequent theories have expanded the social matrix
in which patients' and physicians' roles are situated and provided for
modified models of patients' passivity, they have left intact the original model of the physician-patient relationship as an institutionalized
asymmetrical role set. Thus, physicians' abilities to provide medical
care are assumed to depend on their control over patients.

However, the assumption remains to be tested. Theoretical formulations have said little about *how* physician control is established, nor
have they provided an empirical means of assessing its effects. By and
large, communication between physicians and patients is seen to be
pre-structured by the roles that they play and the obligations attendant to those roles. In short, the communication process is reduced to
a "script" between well-rehearsed actors.

Empirical studies have echoed the theme of asymmetry between
doctors and patients. In part, this is an artifact of the larger issues
such studies address. Investigations of compliance, for example, have
employed various features of verbal interaction to study conditions
under which patients will follow physicians' instructions. Studies of
patient satisfaction, similarly, have treated interaction as a resource
rather than as a topic of research. And many empirical studies of
physician control have completely omitted social interaction from
their research designs, focusing instead on physicians' and patients'
perceptions of communication with one another.

As a body of literature, this research is rife with inconsistent findings. Some of these, as we have seen, result from problems with
method and measurement. However, other empirical contradictions
point to a more serious substantive matter—namely, the very definition of "communication" between physician and patient. Here, as in
theories of the physician-patient relationship, communication is conceptualized as an exchange of information.[5] Thus, "good" communication is seen as the accurate transmission of particular messages.

I have already noted that this definition poses a paradox for theoretical formulations of the physician-patient relationship—namely, that exchange is prohibited when parties to communication processes do not have equal access to the symbolic meaning of information they transmit. To the extent that empirical studies also assume an essential asymmetry between doctors and patients, they too are confronted with a dilemma: If communication is predicated on *symmetrical* relations and the physician-patient relationship is *essentially* asymmetrical, how, then, can doctors and patients communicate with one another?

One step toward resolution of this dilemma is closer examination of what is meant by an "exchange of information." As a first point, we can note that the notion of exchange implies a two-way process, some form of reciprocity in giving and receiving. In order to understand the essential properties of this process, then, one would first need a description of giving and receiving by *both* sides of an exchange. Thus, studies focusing only on physicians' use of "jargon" as a form of information control—without examining patients' responses to it and patients' own use of medical terminology—are insufficient for our purposes.

Secondly, we can note that what "information" consists of is itself unclear. Within a medical setting, for example:

> A patient is most likely to tell the staff those things about himself that he thinks it is important for the staff to know to protect his health. But how does he know what is important? One task of the physician is to educate the patient to report his symptoms properly. The physician does not want the patient telling him everything under the sun. However he *does* want the patient to tell him the significant things. The difficult part is to get the patient to learn which things are significant and which are not. (Roth, 1963a:295)

Ignoring, for the moment, Roth's emphasis on the responsibility of physicians to define important (versus irrelevant) information, we can still see that some sort of definition must be decided upon for routine exchanges of information to occur.

Finally, we can note that "communication" consists of a great deal more information than that which is deliberately told or imparted. The medium of information exchange, whether verbal or nonverbal, can often convey as much information as the content of a message itself. Moreover, media which are heavily used may come to serve purposes other than simple transmission of messages. As Trudgill

(1974) suggests: "Language is not simply a means of communicating information—about the weather or any other subject. It is also a very important means of *establishing and maintaining relationships with other people*" (p. 13; emphasis added). In other words, our social relationships with others are built and sustained through our means of communicating with them.

Whereas much existing work has treated doctor-patient communication as a *by-product* of the physician-patient relationship, Trudgill implies that communication between doctor and patient is really a means of *constituting* that relationship. Following his contention, the study of doctor-patient relations must begin with the empirical investigation of ways in which doctors and patients communicate with one another. Moreover, it must begin with an approach that provides for systematic examination of interaction between doctors and patients as a topic in its own right. The next chapter describes such an approach to collecting naturally occurring encounters in an actual medical setting.

CHAPTER 3

Methods, Measurements, and Medical Encounters

With the likely exception of methodologists, few persons are interested in data collection procedures as topics in and of themselves. As Strong remarks, "Summary descriptions of institutions and rapid surveys of the sources of one's data normally engender a creeping paralysis in the unfortunate reader" (1979:18). Matters of method and measurement are typically found interesting only after a report of some especially provocative set of findings.

Yet it is in the wake of stimulating findings that questions often arise over methodologies employed to produce them. Regarding communication, for example, questions may properly be posed about the identities of participants in discourse, the nature of the settings in which they interact, the channels of communication open to them, the variety of codes mutually available to them, the forms and types of messages they may send, the attitudes expressed through particular messages, the content of messages sent and, finally, the meaning of the interactional events themselves (Hymes, 1964:10; Thorne and Henley, 1975:12–13). As we can see, the substantive significance of any given set of results may be sifted through a finely meshed sieve indeed.

In order to provide readers with a set of coordinates for building their own sieves, this chapter offers an introduction to the setting, participants, and methods used in this study of medical encounters. Through this introduction, I hope to establish both my own warrant for the analyses that follow and a warrant for readers to come to their own informed conclusions about these results.

PROBLEMS OF ACCESS

In 1977 I knew that I wanted to conduct a naturalistic (i.e., uncontrived) study of talk between physicians and patients. I also knew (or, thought I knew) that the chances of collecting systematic observations in a naturalistic medical environment were slim to nonexistent. Obviously, a primary concern in procuring data was the confidentiality of the physician-patient relationship. Whatever transpires between a doctor and patient is ethically and legally regarded as privileged information. Thus, justification for my access to such information became an enormous problem.

Beyond justification, however, lurked the issue of consent. Even if some particular physician or particular set of physicians agreed that a study such as I envisioned *should* be conducted, how could they ethically consent to their own or their patients' unwitting participation in it? And, if I secured consent from individual patients and practitioners, how would I ensure anything more than a haphazard collection of diverse settings, varying medical specialties, and diverse patient symptoms?

Finally, I foresaw difficulties arising in regard to my disciplinary affiliation and standing as an outsider to the medical profession. From a physician's point of view, it seemed that sociologists had had nothing nice to say about medical practice for the past twenty years. For example, one reviewer of *The Unkindest Cut: Life in the Backrooms of Medicine* (Millman, 1977) began his evaluation noting: "During recent years the medical profession in the United States has been inundated by a flood of hate books against physicians. These have varied in type and quality from unsubtle, unjustified vitriolic attacks to thoughtful, well-documented criticisms of the medical establishment and the so-called nonsystem of health care" (Derbyshire, 1977:133). Derbyshire's remarks illuminate more than a few reservations physicians might have about welcoming inquisitive sociologists into their midst.

The numerous trials and tribulations I faced while trying to resolve these problems do not warrant extensive discussion here. Suffice it to say that my solutions entailed certain compromises. These data con-

sist of naturally occurring exchanges between patients and practitioners in training in only one medical specialty—family practice.[1] The
exchanges ensued in the context of only one sort of physician-patient
contact—primary care.[2] And the visits that prompted these exchanges
were all of a single type—ambulatory care encounters.[3] Hence, I
make no claims that generalize my findings to the practices of physicians in different specialties (e.g., obstetrics and gynecology, urology
or general surgery) or patients in different circumstances (e.g., hospitalized or invalid).

However, since ambulatory care encounters constitute a large part
of patients' visits to doctors (i.e., 585 million of over a billion annual
visits), and since patients' frequency of such visits averages nearly
three per year (U.S. Department of Health, Education and Welfare,
1983), these primary care visits are not unrepresentative of encounters in general between patients and their doctors. The physicians in
my study are somewhat atypical, though, as they are practitioners of
one of the newest medical specialties recognized by the American
Medical Association (in 1969).

THE MEDICAL SETTING AND MEDICAL SPECIALTY

Doctors whose encounters I analyze are residents in Family Practice, a medical specialty that requires a three-year-training program
beyond medical school. The program is housed in a family practice
center, which is affiliated with—but located a couple of blocks away
from—a large medical university in the southern United States. The
physicians themselves are from a range of geographical backgrounds:
Of the 45 residents and 6 clinical faculty members who provide patient care, 5 are from the West; 13, from the Midwest; 13, from the
Northeast; and 20, from the Southeast (T. J. Stewart et al., 1980). The
Center has now been in operation for over a decade and is recognized
as an established, well-regarded source of ambulatory patient care
(including emergency, off-hours, laboratory, and x-ray services) for
the community it serves.

The Center provides care for over 6200 active patients, who are
seen on an average of 4.2 visits per year (Pantell et al., 1982). Care is
offered on a fee-for-service basis to patients who are pre-enrolled
there. On pre-enrolling, patients are assigned to individual physicians
(who treat them in about 65 percent of visits).

The sort of care offered by family physicians covers a broad range of patient needs. These physicians are trained in pediatrics, obstetrics and gynecology, internal medicine, surgery, behavioral science, and community medicine, as well as in family medicine itself. As a medical specialty, family practice is unique in at least three important aspects (Lewy, 1977, see also Rakel, 1977). First, residents are trained in "model practice units" (such as the Center), which constitute their primary bases of clinical learning. Within these units, they are responsible for the continuous and comprehensive care of a group of patients who "represent a cross section of the community" (Lewy, 1977:878). Although the primary focus of care is the ambulatory patient, residents are also responsible for those of their patients requiring home or hospital care.

The second distinguishing characteristic of family practice is its inclusion of community medicine into residency training programs. Here, education in epidemiology, biostatistics, occupational and environmental health is stressed, in the belief that "a greater appreciation of the health patterns of the community should lead to a greater understanding of the health needs of the individual" (Lewy, 1977:878–879). Moreover, family physicians are expected to familiarize themselves with the communities in which they practice, rather than leading isolated existences as "scientist-physicians."

The third distinctive ingredient in family practice training is education in the social and behavioral sciences. Curry emphasizes the necessity for including these fields in residents' education for the following reason:

> Medical graduates today usually have a fine background in scientific training. [However] there is an unevenness in the opportunities offered in medical schools to develop critical perceptiveness relating to the emotional aspects of their patients' problems. The recognition and definition of behavioral and emotional problems is more difficult, tedious and time consuming than the discovery of elevated blood pressure or pitting edema . . . time and energy consuming but well worth the price. (Curry, 1979:3)

His description highlights physicians' growing recognition that many patient visits are prompted by matters which are nonmedical. Social, emotional, and behavioral difficulties can also propel patients to their doctors.[4]

Patients are not the only ones seen to benefit by inclusion of social and behavioral materials into family practice curriculums. Bock and Egger (1971) stress the need for family physicians to develop better interpersonal skills and continuing relationships with patients—as individuals, as family members and as citizens in larger communities. Through these means, the practitioner in family practice is expected to become "a personal physician, oriented to the whole patient, who practices both scientific and humanistic medicine" (Statement of the Council on Medical Education, American Medical Association, cited by Lukomnik, 1978:27).[5]

In sum, the popular ideal of a caring physician, devoted to the patient as a "whole person" (rather than to individual body parts), is epitomized in the goals of this specialty. To implement these goals, many training programs now employ technologies that are particularly well suited to social scientific research interests. In facilities such as the Center, for example, "The television camera and microphone in every room, and our behavioral scientists in the monitoring room, have helped enormously" (Curry, 1979:3).

Data Collection

On my first visit to the Center in June 1979, I discovered a setting that seemed to have been especially designed for my purposes.[6] It houses 19 examining rooms, all of which are equipped with high quality ceiling microphones and unobtrusive videocameras located in ceilings' corners. These devices are wired to a remote monitoring room, in which videocassette recorders and video monitors provide unimpeded contact with activities in examining rooms. My problems of access to doctor-patient dialogues were definitely over.

"Informed consent" also dissolved as a hindrance to my study. Since audiotaping and videotaping had been used for several years as part of the training of residents, patients had been exposed to these routinely in the course of receiving care at the Center. During a patient's first visit, the physician responsible for care gives the patient a detailed explanation of the purpose of the recording systems. Then the patient is asked to sign a form which provides his or her informed consent to allow recording for teaching and research purposes.[7] Of course, blanket consent to recording is never solicited. Patients may ask that any particular visit be excepted from recording; they may also exempt themselves from all recording without any effect on their participation in the program. However, patients who do not wish to be recorded at all are few and far between. And, even these patients are given ample opportunity to change their minds, since new consent forms are distributed annually.

The Center's social and behavioral science faculty record patient visits and review them with residents on a regular basis. While residents may request extra video-monitoring sessions (e.g., to gain insight into particularly problematic cases), they may not exempt themselves from routine (i.e., at least once per term) video review by faculty. Since the monitoring sessions are regarded as an essential part of resident training, physician applicants to residencies at the Center are made well aware of their purpose. In fact, some residents claimed that they selected the Center's residency program precisely because of its concern for development of their clinical skills.

Faculty members who monitor the residents are trained in psychology, psychiatry, sociology, social work, and general behavioral science. The diversity of their disciplinary emphases offers residents the chance to obtain multiple perspectives on their own development. For example, a psychologist may be able to offer input on the resident's abilities to make contact with patients who are withdrawn, while a sociologist can give residents insights on their abilities to relate to groups of family members (e.g., in pediatric interviews). Since the American Academy of Family Practice dictates that a set percentage of faculty in any residency training program must be social and behavioral scientists, these nonmedical faculty members and their perspectives are firmly established in the program for resident training. Thus, the third major obstacle to my investigation (my standing as a sociologist and as a nonmedical doctor) was also minimized in this setting. Here I found faculty members—many of whom were themselves social scientists—who were already receptive to such analyses as I proposed.

Over the course of my ten-week visit to the Center, monitoring faculty members assisted my collection of 21 videotaped two-party exchanges between adult patients (i.e., 16 years or older) and family physicians. Since several of the faculty were independently interested in physician-parent-child exchanges, and since two-party talk was the simplest point of departure for conversation analysis, I excluded pediatric visits from my corpus of materials.

Patients in my collection of exchanges range in age from 16 to 82 years. They come from a variety of backgrounds, including those of professional, domestic, construction worker, and unemployed carpenter. Of the 20 patients, 5 were black females; 6, white females; 4, black males; and 5, white males (see Note 5, Chapter 1).

Physicians in these exchanges are residents in the program, who are typically in their late twenties or early thirties.[8] Seventeen of the exchanges involve male physicians and four involve female physicians (see below). All of the doctors are white.

Because these interactions occurred during actual physician visits, they are not standardized according to duration of exchange, purpose of visit, or length of relationship between doctor and patient. Some physicians and patients had known one another for three years at the time of recording, while others were meeting for the first time. Some visits were routine checks of long-standing problems; others uncovered new complaints. Although all residents had patient visits scheduled for at least one half hour intervals, some visits took less than 30 minutes and some took considerably more.

By now the reader should have a clear picture of one compromise necessitated by my mode of data collection, namely the lack of a standardized or random sample. Actual taping of these encounters was conducted for purposes of resident training rather than sociological analysis. Thus, I had no control over who was to be taped with whom. For example, I include a total of 21 separate exchanges in my data collection. But of these, 18 involve different physician residents, while 3 track the same resident over the course of his morning's patient rounds. So, I can provide a relatively detailed portrayal of variations in physician's responses to patients for one doctor, but not for all the doctors included in my collection.

Further, these materials include 14 exchanges with white male physicians and 4 with white female physicians. Hence, although patients are Black in 9 of the 21 dyads, no Black physician is included in my collection.[9] And the 4 white female physicians in these encounters were among the first cohort (i.e., group of more than two) ever to begin training at the Center. Proportionate to their numbers, then, women physicians are overrepresented in my sample.

Although these constitute important limitations in my data (to be considered further in subsequent chapters), they do not present the same problems that they might for another sort of investigation. If this study were conducted to analyze characteristics of physicians or those of patients, my data would be inadequate for generalizing beyond those doctors and patients included in my collection. However, as I explained in Chapter 1, my purposes are somewhat different. As my point of departure, I take it that certain local technical problems arise for physicians and patients *whenever* the two interact. Such tasks as opening up a state of talk, maintaining an ordered exchange, or terminating interaction must be accomplished on an ongoing basis regardless of the identities of the physicians and patients involved. Thus, the orderliness and stability of patterns of interaction between physicians and patients are seen as products of interactional problems—problems that must be resolved wherever doctors and patients meet for purposes of conducting an exchange.[10] Accordingly, my analyses begin with the detailed examination of interaction itself, in taped and transcribed records.

TRANSCRIBING

Transcribing interaction for the purposes of analyzing the very structure of interaction is a time-consuming process. Over the course of my ten weeks at the Center, my actual data collection took very little time in comparison to the task of transcribing. The 21 two-party exchanges yielded 532 typed pages of transcript. However, there was no way around this job. Conversation analysis takes the tapes and transcripts as its raw materials, rather than as means to an end.

Although researchers who do interviews may ignore "background noise" (e.g., laughter or audible exhalations), and may neglect variations in such things as pitch or amplitude, conversation analysts attempt to include all such matters in their transcripts (West and Zimmerman, 1982:515–518). For them, transcribing is properly part of analysis itself, rather than a subsidiary chore to be assigned a secretary or trained assistant. A first principle of such analysis is that the details of *how* something is said (in a whisper, in a shout, with a stutter, with a drawl, etc.) can be as important as the content of talk itself (see especially Jefferson and Schegloff, 1975). Jefferson, a pioneer in the field, describes its aim as follows: "A task we have undertaken is to provide transcripts that not only serve for current research interests, but are 'research generative.' This means in its best sense that the transcripts, by capturing events, illuminate possible features of the data which are not yet known to be features; and at least that they *preserve* for future investigation, such as-yet-unknown orderly features" (1971:1). To would-be conversation analysts, struggling to discriminate inhalations from exhalations, or "eh-heh-heh's" from "heh-eh-heh's" (both streams of laughter particles), the task may seem akin to that of field ethnographers who are impossibly instructed to "capture everything" in their field notes. Inasmuch as both forms of analysis are involved in discovering organization and organizing principles, their aims are in fact comparable. The analysis of *how* persons achieve orderly talk—like that of social organization of any other sort—is best conducted through meticulous examination of their actual behavior in its natural context (for related approaches to nonverbal behavior, see Ekman, 1980; Kendon, 1981; Scheflen, 1972; Scherer and Ekman, 1982).

A major issue generated by these concerns surrounds the practice of "normalizing" speakers' utterances. For transcribers of interviews, interrogations, and the like, "normalization" is generally regarded as the practice of translating what was heard on tape into grammatically "proper" language. Mishler offers the following observations on this practice:

> Clearly, a range of phenomena that are integral to naturally-occurring speech have no analogue on the printed page, at least in its standard familiar form. Omitted from the great variety of printed texts such as newspaper reports, fictional and nonfictional narratives, and scientific papers, even when they include quotations, are such features of speech as intonation, pitch, pacing, volume, filled and unfilled pauses, nonlexical vocalizations, false starts, repetitions, interruptions and overlaps between speakers. These omissions are particularly noticeable when the text is presumed to represent speech, as in transcripts of journalistic or research interviews, of courtroom testimony, and of committee hearings. (1984: Chapter 2, p. 3)

In "textualized" versions of speech, then, we find speakers' utterances become hypercorrect, even abnormal—"normalized" to delete precisely those characteristics which distinguish speech from text (see also Cicourel, 1975).

To illuminate the hazards involved with this practice, consider but one feature of naturally occurring speech that is obliterated by normalization—*repetition* of prior utterances. In the variety of texts noted by Mishler (newspaper reports, narratives, and scientific papers), utterances appear according to an economy that allocates only one per speaker. Thus, instances of speakers repeating (or partially repeating) the same utterance twice are deleted from the text. Deletion is also the fate of utterances that constitute repetition of what another party has just said.

However, Jefferson and her colleagues note that repetition of utterances can accomplish a range of interactional ends. For example, Jefferson and Schegloff (1975) observe that two parties speaking simultaneously may engage in competition for the floor by recycling portions of their own talk over the ongoing speech of another party (transcribing conventions used throughout this book are presented at the front of this book, pp. xiii–xiv; here, brackets indicate the onset of simultaneous speech):

```
Ken:   No, they're women who'v devo ⎡ded their-
Roger:                                ⎣They're women that hadda =

Roger:   ⎧⎛bad love ⎛life 'n became nuns.hh ⎛heh hh!
       = ⎨⎜
Ken:     ⎩⎝their-   ⎝their life-             ⎝their life, to uh
                      ‾‾‾‾‾‾‾‾‾‾
                         (0.6)
Ken:        the devotion of the church.
```

(Jefferson and Schegloff, 1975:11)

In this fragment, we see Ken recycling components of previously produced talk ("their- their- their life-") over Roger's continuing stream of talk, thus preserving a few words ("the devotion of the church") for production in the clear.

Elsewhere, Schegloff, Jefferson, and Sacks (1977) observe that *repairs* of another party's trouble-source turn may be initiated by partially repeating components of that turn:

```
A:  Well Monday, lemme think. Monday, Wenesday, an'
    Fridays I'm home by one ten.
B:  One ten?
A:  Two o'clock. My class ends one ten.
```

(Schegloff et al., 1977:368)

Here, for example, we see B's repetition ("One ten?") of A's estimated time of arrival elicits a subsequent modification by A ("Two o'clock. My class ends one ten."). Obviously such finely detailed observations and subsequent analyses are completely obscured in transcribed exchanges that read like the script for a play.

The lesson for transcribers is that every effort must be made to preserve the sounds that are heard on tape (or viewed, in the case of video) in the transcripts themselves, even when those sounds are not immediately intelligible to the listener. On hearing ambiguous sounds (e.g., noises that might be transcribed in more than one way), conversation analysts will indicate the ambiguities in the transcripts themselves. Even with these precautions, Jefferson warns that there is no guarantee that the transcripts alone will suffice for unspecified research tasks; they are properly employed as an adjunct to the tape-recorded materials (see "Transcribing Conventions Used in the Text," pp. xiii–xiv).

In one particular area, these dicta pose a problem for analysts of doctor-patient interaction. Verbatim transcripts involve the faithful rendition of spoken names, places, and personal identities. This practice evolved through a concern for "lost" data and "lost" research problems, due to *non*verbatim transcription. An example is provided by Jefferson's overview of difficulties associated with the use of pseudonyms:

> Agnes: Thirdy sevin years ago tuhni::ght we were on ar way tuh
> Ventura.
> Guy: Hm. Wuddiyuh know about that.
> Agnes: Sanna BARBRA hhh huh//huh
> Guy: BARBRA. Uh huh,
> Agnes: We gotta MARIAN did'n we.
> Guy: Mmyuh.

(Jefferson, 1971:5)

In this fragment, the name *Marian* has been used as a pseudonym for *Barbara*, the real name of the couple's daughter. Hence, what was actually an artfully conducted nameplay on people and places (going to Santa Barbara and getting Barbara) is "lost" by using *Marian* as a pseudonym for the daughter's name. The point, notes Jefferson (1971), is that names in themselves are interactional resources for speakers' use, which the substitution of pseudonyms completely obscures.

However, the use of real names in public transcripts of physician-patient discourse would constitute a breach of the confidentiality assumed by the doctor-patient relationship. Indeed, one purpose of my ten-week visit at the Center was conversion of the tapes (which could not leave the premises) into transcripts (which could), in order to protect the rights to privacy of those physicians and patients involved in my collection of exchanges. In the chapters which follow, identifying references to places and parties involved have been disguised, and I offer fragments for the reader's inspection only when speakers' anonymity is ensured.

With this exception, I have endeavored to present transcripts that pay strictest attention to representing what was heard *as it was heard* in fine detail. The job was time-consuming and painstaking, assuredly (it easily requires eight to ten hours of time to transcribe each hour of audiotape; the ratio increases considerably with video). But, as I hope to demonstrate in the chapters that follow, the time and energy involved in such work are more than repaid by its potential rewards.

Ethnographic Insights

Prior to closing this discussion of methods and measurements, it is only fitting that I offer a few words on my own experiences while engaging in this research. During my stay at the Center I got to know many of the medical faculty and residents fairly well. As a visitor, of course, it is always easier to strike up friendships in a limited time period. But various house-sitting (and animal-care) arrangements I exchanged for accommodations also facilitated a closer, perhaps more humane, means of establishing contact than might otherwise exist in a research setting. As a result, I developed many collegial relationships and some close friendships among the faculty and residents at the Center.

Undeniably, these associations have had an impact on my research. Some issues I might never have addressed arose first in casual conversations with faculty members (discussing patterns I had observed on the tapes). Other topics emerged after listening to residents comment on particular difficulties they encounter in certain sorts of patient contacts. Too, after ten weeks spent launching my analyses in the Center itself, I am sure that my sensitivities to the data are different than they might have been if I had merely received the recordings by mail. So I have in some degree opened myself up to the subjective perspective of physicians in these exchanges. And I have developed a healthy respect for the constraints on physicians' time, energy, and capacities for empathy imposed by the day-to-day demands of clinical practice.

However, strange as it may seem, I also feel a very special attachment to those patients who participated in the exchanges I analyze. We have never met, of course; I have never come face-to-face with any of the patients recorded in this collection. Still, the privileged access I had to intimate details of their lives forged a kind of closeness that makes these limitations seem trivial. On one tape, a very painful interaction was recorded between a female physician and a male patient who had beaten his wife. As I transcribed each of the physician's and patient's utterances, I could not help but be moved by the distress evidenced in their interaction with one another. Another exchange, between a male physician and a female patient, contains a story (told for the first time, says the patient) of the patient having been molested by her stepfather when she was only eight years old. The patient was understandably devastated by the experience, and I was doubly devastated while watching and listening to the tape. Prior to viewing these encounters, I had never imagined the full range of human experiences that may unfold between physician and patient.

Strictly speaking, this research is not ethnographic in nature. My analyses focus on observable conversational events, and do not include the motivations, predispositions, or ulterior motives that may be in the minds of those involved. Hence, relationships I formed with participants in the setting do not pose quite the same problems for my analysis that they might for field ethnographers. For example:

> In some settings the special kind of witnessing which is the essence of most fieldwork—the detached and analytical perspective, the gathering and recording of concrete detail to be sifted into analytic reports which will circulate to outsiders—may feel like a particular violation (Hughes, 1971:505). Groups demanding extreme commitment and partisanship may not want the presence of an avowed neutral; parties and other sociable occasions presume expressiveness, unseriousness, and suspension of consequentiality—tacit rules which conflict with the instrumental attitudes and tasks involved in doing a field study. (Thorne, 1980:289)

Since the subjective perspectives of participants are not my objects of inquiry in this study, I did not run the risk of coloring descriptions of those perspectives by developing ties to participants.

However, the weeks I spent fully immersed in the activities of the Center itself—sitting out in the waiting area with patients, monitoring patients in examining rooms while waiting for doctors to appear, attending lunchtime grand rounds with physicians, and living, for one month, with a new resident and his wife—all are experiences which have helped me develop a more complete picture of the larger scale of activities in which my physician-patient exchanges are situated. Throughout the chapters to follow, my analyses are conducted with appreciation of these larger contexts.

THE APPROACH TO DATA

The claim to be involved in research on such things as medical misunderstandings may seem incongruous in the company of my explicit disavowal of interest in the "subjective perspectives" of participants in this study. Ordinarily, "understandings," "agreements," and "consensuses" are thought to lie properly within the domain of research on socially constructed meanings (e.g., Emerson, 1970; Ball, 1967; Becker et al., 1961; Berger and Luckman, 1966; Freidson, 1961). However, as noted earlier, studies of socially constructed meanings have told us little about the organization of interaction used to produce those meanings. For example, in a study cited earlier (see Chapter 2) Emerson (1970) observes:

> Medical talk stands for and continually expresses allegiance to the medical definition. . . . The special language found in staff-patient contacts contributes to depersonalization and desexualization of the encounter. . . . The definite article replaces the pronoun adjective in reference to body parts, so that [in gynecological visits] the doctor refers to "the vagina" and never "your vagina." (p. 81)

In inviting us to attend to the substitution of definite articles for personal pronouns, Emerson illustrates one of the ways in which depersonalization permeates the interaction between gynecologist and patient. But the principles governing the construction of depersonalized talk are not addressed in her study. Thus, we learn little about the topical contexts in which definite articles are introduced, the conversational events that trigger their introductions, or the ways in which patients' speech responds to the depersonalized realities constructed by their physicians.

Elsewhere (West and Zimmerman, 1982), I propose that conversation analysis differs from ethnographic analysis in its explicit focus on the *systematics* of producing utterances, sequences of utterances, and other nonverbal expressions.[11] These systematics (e.g., of turn-taking, of repair, or of coordinating gaze with utterance productions) can in turn furnish the framework for analyzing (1) the ways in which conversational events achieve a particular meaning or delineated range of alternative meanings in a situated context; (2) the ways in which these events contribute to, establish, negotiate, or expose a definition or definitions of the situation; and (3) the ways in which these events warrant statements regarding participants' states of mind, motives, feelings, and so on. However, the concern of conversation analysis is not with the psychological processes internal to participants in interaction, nor merely with the meanings given to situations by individual participants:

> The concern instead is this: Insofar as *members* recognize and respond to such objects as "state of mind" or "motive" or "the meaning of a situation," [we take it that] such objects are methodically produced and appreciated *by members,* an achievement in need of description and analysis in its own right. (West and Zimmerman, 1982:511)

The point worth emphasizing here is that this approach to interactional data does not originate in any desire to capture participants' "subjective perspectives" of their situations (Sacks, 1963, p. 7, n. 7). This very notion is often interpreted commonsensically, as meaning "getting into someone's mind," or gaining access to their private thoughts and intentions. But Sacks proposes that adoption of participants' "subjective perspectives" entails conceiving of the subject matter in a particular way, especially in terms of certain methodological constraints on the identification of structures in participants' talk or behavior. So, not any patterned activity uncovered by analysis is legitimately a feature of the social organization of activities being studied. The conversation analyst must furnish a warrant for claiming that an observed regularity is one produced *by* and *for* the "appreciation and use by co-participants" *from the observable data of conversational activities* (Schegloff and Sacks, 1974:234; emphases added).[12]

SUMMARY AND CONCLUSIONS

The purpose of this chapter has been to introduce readers to these data and the procedures for collecting them. As we have seen, the family physicians involved in these exchanges are completing their residencies in a relatively new field of medicine. Hence, they are neither longtime practitioners, nor are they comparable in medical specialty to doctors included in many previous studies of doctor-patient communication (cf. Korsch et al., 1968; Fisher, 1983; Tannen and Wallat, 1983; Wallen et al., 1979). To the extent that these factors are likely to influence my results, it is probably safe to surmise that their influence lies in a conservative direction. For example, these physicians are in a training program which emphasizes the impor-tance of communication skills, and in a specialty dedicated to per-sonal, comprehensive, continuous care and the humanistic practice of medicine.

But my corpus of materials does not constitute a random sample of physicians, patients, or doctor-patient exchanges. My lack of control over such variables as length of interaction or degree of acquaintance between doctor and patient resulted in a nonstandardized final collec-tion, which includes exchanges of various lengths between doctors and patients with different past contacts. Thus, generalizations based on my findings cannot be extended to physicians, patients, or doctor-patient exchanges at large.

What are generalizable are the trans-situational problems of con-ducting interaction between two people on the occasion of visits to the doctor. The orderly exchange of turns at talk, the organization of questions and answers, the resolution of potential mishearings and misunderstandings, and the integration of sociable commentary into instrumental discourse must all be managed on those particular oc-casions on which physicians and patients interact. The systematic pro-cedures used to resolve these problems are my subjects of analysis in the next chapters.

CHAPTER 4

Turn-Taking in Doctor-Patient Dialogues*

Turn-taking is used for the ordering of moves in games, for allocating political office, for regulating traffic at intersections, for serving customers at business establishments, and for talking in interviews. . . . It is obviously a prominent type of social organization, one whose instances are implicated in a wide range of other activities. (Sacks, Schegloff and Jefferson, 1974:696)

Whatever else transpires in physicians' interactions with patients must somehow be reconciled with the organization of their turns at talk. To date, such activities as history taking, examination, diagnosis and treatment have not yet been consigned to computers.[1] Hence, performance of these tasks relies largely on the face-to-face exchange of speech between doctors and their patients.

In everyday life, we appear to recognize the significance of orderly speech exchange for attainment of conversational goals. Getting across the content of a message often seems contingent on such matters as being able to get a word in edgewise, sustaining a train of thought without interruption, and receiving some indication that one's conversational partners are in fact listening.

But little attention has been paid to the implications of talk's turn-taking organization for participants in medical encounters. Part of the neglect may stem from an overemphasis on the importance of

*A preliminary report of findings here presented is titled "When the Doctor is a Lady: Power, Status and Gender in Physician-Patient Encounters," *Symbolic Interaction* 7 (1984): 87–106.

physicians' contributions to these exchanges. Physicians are, after all, the ones to perform examinations, issue diagnoses, and formulate "orders" for treatment. However, insofar as such tasks are dependent on patients' contributions to talk (e.g., expressing concerns, reporting symptoms, or indicating "where it hurts"), physicians' performance of their clinical work is ultimately contingent on the ordering of their talk with patients.

Elsewhere, the substance of spoken interaction is found to be a fundamental means of ordering social activities and organizing social relationships. For example, there is now an extensive body of research suggesting that males interrupt females far more often than the reverse, across a variety of situations (Argyle et al., 1968; Eakins and Eakins, 1976; McMillan et al., 1977; Natale et al., 1979; Octigan and Niederman, 1979; Willis and Williams, 1976). Findings of my own earlier work indicate that males' interruptions of females in cross-sex conversations constitute an exercise of power and control over their conversational partners (Zimmerman and West, 1975; West and Zimmerman, 1977; West, 1979; 1982; West and Zimmerman, 1983).

Of course, power is an important facet of many other social relationships, such as those between whites and Blacks, bosses and employees, and—of particular interest here—doctors and patients. Recall Parsons's perspective on the matter, summarized by Wolinsky (1980): "The practitioner must have control over the interaction with the patient, ensuring that the patient will comply with the prescribed regimen" (p. 163). Insofar as the physician-patient relationship is, as some have contended, *essentially* asymmetrical by our cultural standards, it is here that we would expect to find highlighted the dynamics of micropolitical exchange, through, among other things, a greater proportion of interruptions initiated by superordinate parties to talk:

> In front of, and defending the political-economic structure that determines our lives and defines the context of human relationships, there is the micropolitical structure that helps maintain it. This micropolitical structure is the substance of our everyday experience. The humiliation of being a subordinate is often felt most sharply and painfully when one is ignored or interrupted while speaking, towered over or forced to move by another's bodily presence, or cowed unknowingly into dropping the eyes, the head, the shoulders. (Henley, 1977:3)

In this chapter, I report results of my analysis of the organization of turn-taking between patients and family physicians. My preliminary findings offer some empirical support for the archetypal relationship thought to exist between doctors and patients: Physicians interrupt patients far more often than the reverse, *except* when the doctor is a "lady." Then, I find that gender seems to have a greater impact than professional status where women physicians are concerned. Consideration of these results leads me to address such issues as the respective parts played by power, status, and gender in social interaction.

Since interruptions constitute a type of transition between speaker turns, my point of departure is the model of turn-taking in conversation developed by Harvey Sacks, Emanuel Schegloff, and Gail Jefferson (1974) which furnishes a systematic approach to speaker alternation in naturally occurring speech exchange.

THE MODEL

Sacks et al. (1974) observe that speech exchange systems in general are arranged to ensure that (1) one party talks at a time and (2) speaker change recurs. These features are seen to normatively organize a variety of forms of talk, including casual conversation, formal debate, and high ceremony. Conversation is distinguished from other forms of exchange by its variable distributions of turn size, turn order and turn content (for further discussion of doctor-patient discourse as conversation, see Chapter 5).

Within this framework, a turn at talk consists not merely of the temporal duration of an utterance but of the right and obligation to speak which is allocated to a particular speaker. Turns are built out of what Sacks et al. term "unit-types," consisting of possibly complete words, phrases, clauses or sentences, depending on their context. Further, unit-types are described as "projective" devices, in that they allow enough information prior to their completion to allow the hearer to anticipate an upcoming transition place. In other words, the end of a possibly complete unit-type is the proper place for transition to occur between speaker turns.

My prior research has led me to distinguish between two general categories of simultaneous speech: *overlaps* (briefly, errors in transition timing) and *interruptions* (violations of speaker turns).[2] Overlaps are defined as stretches of simultaneous speech initiated by a "next" speaker just as the current speaker arrives at a possible transition

place (Zimmerman and West, 1975:113–115). Jefferson and Schegloff (1975) note that such instances of simultaneity are common
where the current speaker stretches or drawls the final syllable of an
utterance, or adds a tag-question to an otherwise complete statement:

(Dyad 19:305–307)[3]

    Patient: I li:ve better and so I- they don' bo:ther me
                too mu:ch, ⌈y'know?⌉

    Physician: ⌊O::kay.⌋

Here (as indicated by the brackets), the physician starts her "Okay"
just at what would ordinarily be the proper completion point for the
patient's utterance ("They don't bother me too much"). However, the
patient's addition of a tag-question ("Y'know?") results in their colli-
sion. I regard such an instance of simultaneous speech as a possible
error in transition timing rather than as an indication that the physician is not listening. Indeed, one must listen very carefully in order
to anticipate the upcoming completion of a current speaker's utterance and begin speaking precisely on cue, with no silence intervening
between turns.

A related form of simultaneity "provoked" by careful listening is
what Jefferson (1973) terms a "display of independent knowledge."
For example, "saying the same thing at the same time" as someone
else indicates not only that one is attending to them, but also that one
is listening carefully enough to predict what they are going to say:

(Dyad 1:325–331)

    Physician: An::d Ornade ha:s one called isopropamide iodide,
                an:d it ha:s uh, phenylpropanolamine an':: Neosy-
                nephrine ⌈Ye:ah it's a small amount- it's not that-⌉
    Patient: ⌊So it- a small amount's but not that-⌋ =
    Patient: = Right =
    Physician: = It's six of one und half a doz ⌈en a the⌉ o:ther.
    Patient: ⌊Uh-huh⌋

In this excerpt, for example, just as the physician says "It's a small
amount, it's not that" the patient independently produces the same

thing—thus displaying her careful attention to both the form and content of the physician's emerging utterance.

In contrast, the fragment below illustrates an instance of interruption. An interruption is an initiation of simultaneous speech which intrudes deeply into the internal structure of a current speaker's utterance; operationally, it is found more than a syllable away from a possibly complete unit-type's boundaries (Zimmerman and West, 1975:113–115). Unlike overlaps or displays of independent knowledge, interruptions have no rationale for their occurrence in considerations of active listening (e.g., concerns for minimizing silence between speaker turns or displaying independent understanding). In fact, inasmuch as the rules for turn-taking assign the turnspace to the current speaker until a possible turn-transition point is reached (Sacks et al., 1974:706), an interrupting speaker is engaged in *violation of the current speaker's right* to be engaged in speaking. The following excerpt offers an illustration of the potential effects of such intrusion:

(Dyad 1:945–954)

((Here, the physician and patient have been discussing the
effectiveness of sleeping pills when used over an extended
time period. The physician argues that the patient will be
better off doing without such medication; the patient argues
that her anxieties over a forthcoming trip will interfere
with her effectiveness on the job for which the trip is to
be taken.))

Physician: . . . prob'ly settle dow:n gradjully, a little
           bit, once yuh get used to it. =
Patient: = The- press:: ⌈ure's gonna-
Physician: ⌊Well if it doe::sn',
Physician: Secobar:bital's not gonna help.
                       (.2)
Patient: We:ll,
                       (.2)
Physician: It's gonna make things worse.

The physician's intrusion ("Well if it doesn', Secobarbital's not gonna help") occurs where the patient is nowhere near completion of her utterance, and the patient drops out almost instantly, leaving her

utterance hanging incomplete. As I note in the preface to this fragment, this physician and patient had been arguing about whether or
not he ought to issue her a prescription for sleeping pills. One might
imagine that his exasperation with the argument might have
prompted him to cut off the patient's protests, especially since this
patient was requesting refills for sixteen other medications (including
Valium and Serax) prior to departing on her trip. However, the
method used by the doctor to superimpose his opinion over that of the
patient is interruption of her turn at talk, that is, violation of her
speaking right. Later in this chapter, I will focus on the content of
such interruptions between speakers in the physician-patient exchanges in my collection.

INTERRUPTIONS IN MEDICAL DIALOGUES

Instances of simultaneous speech were first located in the 532 pages
of transcribed exchanges. Using the criteria specified in the preceding discussion, I separated instances of interruption (i.e., deep intrusions into the internal structure of speakers' utterances) from other
types of simultaneity. Then I compared the initiations of interruptions by physician and patient in each dyad in the collection.[4]

Recall Parsons' suggestion that the physician-patient relationship is
essentially an asymmetrical one. Distributions of physician-initiated
and patient-initiated interruptions would lend support to such a
claim.

Inspecting Table 1, we see that a total of 188 instances of interruption occurred. Of these, physicians initiated 67 percent (126) and
patients initiated 33 percent (62). Thus, doctors interrupted patients
far more often than vice versa. Interruptions display further patterned asymmetries according to patients' race and gender. For example, the ratios of physicians' interruptions to patients' interruptions
are: 1.1 (or nearly equal) for white male patients; 1.8 for white female
patients; 2.6 for Black male patients; and 4.4 for Black female patients. Moreover, in the two dyads characterized by more patient-
initiated than physician-initiated interruption (those to which foot-
notes 1 and 2 are appended), the patient is hard of hearing on the
one hand, and mentally retarded on the other. With the exception of
these exchanges, doctors interrupted patients more in every dialogue

TABLE 1
Interruptions in Encounters between Patients and Male Physicians

	Percentage of Physician Interruptions		*Percentage of Patient Interruptions*	
Black female patient, 16 years	91	(10)	9	(1)
Black female patient, 20 years	100	(1)	—	(0)
Black female patient, 31 years	77	(20)	23	(6)
White female patient, 17 years	100	(1)	—	(0)
White female patient, 32 years	67	(10)	33	(5)
White female patient, 36 years	69	(11)	31	(5)
White female patient, 53 years	73	(29)	27	(11)
White female patient, 58 years	80	(4)	20	(1)
White female patient, 82 years[1]	37	(7)	63	(12)
Black male patient, 17 years	56	(5)	44	(4)
Black male patient, 26 years	100	(7)	—	(0)
Black male patient, 36 years	67	(4)	33	(2)
White male patient, 16 years	100	(1)	—	(0)
White male patient, 16 years	67	(2)	33	(1)
White male patient, 31 years	60	(3)	40	(2)
White male patient, 36 years	58	(7)	42	(5)
White male patient, 56 years[2]	36	(4)	64	(7)
TOTAL	67	(126)	33	(62)

1. This patient is hard of hearing.
2. This patient is mentally retarded.

in this group. However, this group is comprised only of interchanges between patients and *male* physicians.

Table 2 presents the distribution of interruptions between patients and *female* physicians. And in this case we can see that the statistical asymmetries depicted in Table 1 are exactly reversed. Whereas male physicians (in the aggregate) contribute 67 percent of all interruptions relative to their patients' 33 percent, female physicians (in the aggregate) initiate only 32 percent of interruptions relative to their patients' 68 percent. Moreover, patients in exchanges with female physicians interrupt as much or more than their physicians in each dyad in this collection.

Although the group of exchanges involving women doctors contains only four dyads, it is at least worth noting that the two interac-

TABLE 2

Interruptions in Encounters between
Patients and Female Physicians

	Percentage of Physician Interruptions	Percentage of Patient Interruptions
Black female patient, 52 years	50 (7)	50 (7)
Black female patient, 67 years	40 (6)	60 (9)
Black male patient, 58 years	28 (5)	72 (13)
White male patient, 38 years	8 (1)	92 (11)
TOTAL	32 (19)	68 (40)

tions that approximate symmetrical relationships between the parties
involved (the first two listed in Table 2) are same-sex exchanges between women doctors and women patients. These symmetries are
more striking when one considers the differences in race and age
between them (the patients in both dyads are Black and the physicians
are white; the patients are both considerably older than their physicians). My earlier research on same-sex exchanges between white females conversing in public places also suggested that casual
conversation between females tend to display symmetrical distributions of interruptions.

Obviously, the variety of race, age, and gender combinations in a
sample of this size precludes extensive extrapolation regarding the
composite effects of these factors. There is, for example, only one
white male patient engaged in an exchange with a white female physician; similarly, there is only one sixty-seven-year-old patient involved in talk with a physician of half her years. Still, the consistency
of patterns of physician and patient-initiated interruption displayed
in Tables 1 and 2 offers some empirical evidence for the asymmetrical
relationship posited between physicians and patients—*except* when the
doctor is a "lady."

As noted in Chapter 2, Parsons's analysis constitutes a theoretical
formulation of this relationship, rather than an empirical description
of it. Thus, he provides merely an ideal type with which empirical
findings may be compared. These data offer support for his views
where male physicians are concerned. Insofar as interruptions constitute violations of persons' rights to be engaged in speaking, there is
ample evidence in the transcripts that patients' rights to speak are
systematically and disproportionately violated by their male doctors.
However, when physicians are women, the asymmetrical relationship

between doctor and patient is exactly reversed: the posited asymmetry is stood on its head when women doctors are involved. In order to discuss the implications of these results, I move now to consider the relationship between asymmetrical patterns of interruption and interactional control.

Conversational Dominance

In previously comparing conversations between men and women and exchanges between parents and children, I suggested that males' use of interruptions might display dominance or control to females (and to any witnesses), just as parents' interruptions communicated aspects of parental control to children and to others present (West and Zimmerman, 1977:527). If patients can be likened to children (as claimed by Parsons and Fox, 1952), then we might regard the violations of their speaking rights by male physicians as displays of the physicians' interactional control. Parsons's contention was that patients' situational dependency on physicians, physicians' professional prestige, and their authority over patients all ensure physicians the necessary leverage for controlling interpersonal encounters. But, if physicians' control is to be exerted in actual dialogues with patients, one would expect some ready vehicle might be available in any medical exchange for demonstrating the physician's power.

While medical sociologists place heavy emphasis on social roles as determinants of behavior, the actual behaviors of persons in social roles remain to be enacted in everyday life. In short, such scripts as may exist for the physician-patient encounter must always be negotiated on the basis of situational exigencies. However, as Zimmerman notes:

> It would surely be odd if a society were designed so that its institutions were partly constructed of role-relationships, but lacked any systematic mechanism for articulating societal roles within the features of various interactional settings. . . . [And] stranger still if this articulation were itself not socially organized. Strangest of all would be a state of affairs in which the instantiation of a role in an actual situation had no bearing on the understanding of roles in general, or the sense of "objectivity" and transcendence of the role. (Zimmerman, 1978:12)

His observations invite us to look more closely at the ways in which the respective roles of patient and doctor might be played out in the organization of actual interactions between the two.

Hence, rather than regarding the physician's authority as super-imposed onto encounters with patients in "well-rehearsed," script-like fashion (cf. Wilson, 1970), we must examine the dynamics of actual medical exchanges to see how power and control are constituted between participants in those exchanges. A telling example is offered by the fragment used earlier to demonstrate the potential effects of interruption itself. There, a disagreement between a (white male) physician and (white female) patient was ultimately resolved by the doctor's interruption of the patient's opinion (regarding sleeping pills) with his own contrary opinion ("They won't help"). In that excerpt we saw interruption used to advance the physician's (expert) perspective while simultaneously cutting off the patient's (lay) point of view.

Another example of the relationship between interruptions and interactional dominance was furnished by a friend—in this case, a male physician. Prior to writing up the results of this analysis, I discussed with him the tendency of male physicians to interrupt patients in these encounters. My friend did not find this trend a surprising one, and explained, "That's because so many patients are still answering your last question when you're trying to ask them the *next* one!" His "explanation" was of interest for two reasons. First, it fails as an explanation on the grounds that answers follow questions, not the other way around. Hence, a speaker interrupting an answer with a "next question" is disavowing the obligation to listen to the answer to a prior question (see Chapter 5). But second, my doctor-friend's explanation was of empirical interest, since I had already begun to notice that a great many physician-initiated interruptions in these data were composed of doctors' questions to their patients.

Consider the following fragment, which shows the staccato pace at which physicians' "next" questions can follow their "last" ones:

(Dyad 20:053–074)

> Patient: It us:ually be (1.0) ((she reaches down to
>   touch her calf with her left hand)) i:n he:ah.
>   You: know, it jus' [be a li:l-
> Physician: [Can y' pull up] yer cuff there
>   for me? (.6) Duh yuh have the <u>pain</u> right <u>no::w</u>?
>   (.2)

    Patient: Um-um. No, it ⌈ha::ppens   ⌉
    Physician: ⌊It's not happ'ning right now::?⌋
    Patient: ss-°some- Only one: time when ah w ⌈as heah.⌉
    Physician: ⌊Can y⌋ uh take
          yer shoe: off for me please?
                    (.8)
          ((Patient removes her shoe))
    Patient: ⌈But I- ⌉
    Physician: ⌊WHU:⌋ :T'RE YUH DO::ING, when yuh no:dice the
          pai:n
                    (.4)
          ((Physician bends over to touch the muscles in the
          patient's legs))
    Patient: We:ll, I thi:nk that- Well, so:metime I jus' be si:ttin'
          theah. (1.0) An' yih: know: ih ji:st- (1.2) ((she shrugs,
          holding up both palms)) Then I fee:l a liddul pai:n in
          theah. (.2) Yih know, ji:st- gra:dually (.4) It
          gradually c ⌈ome o:n.   ⌉
    Physician: ⌊Take thi:s⌋ shoe: off?

We can note here that each of the physician's intrusions into his (Black female) patient's turn at talk is patently reasonable and warranted by the external constraints of medical examination and treatment. To ask where a patient is feeling pain, how often, when, or under what conditions is all justified by, even required for, precise diagnosis of a problem (cf. Cicourel, 1975; 1978). However, when these inquiries cut off what the patient is in the process of saying, particularly when what she is saying is presumably the necessary response to a "prior" needed question, then the physician is not only violating the patient's rights to speak, but he is also systematically cutting off potentially valuable information *on which he must himself rely* to achieve a diagnosis (see also Frankel, 1984).[5]

Just below, a similar pattern is evident:

(Dyad 2:085–099)

((Here, the doctor is inquiring about a recent injury to the patient's back caused by an auto accident.))

    Patient: When I'm sitting upright. Y'know =
    Physician: = More so than it was even before?

Patient: Yay::es =

Physician: = Swelling 'r anything like that thet chew've
             no:ticed?

                             (.)

Patient: Nuh:o, not the ⌈t I've nodi-
                                ⌊TEN:::DER duh the tou⌋ ch? press:ing
Physician:
             any?

Patient: No::, jus' when it's- si::tting.

Physician: Okay: =

Patient   = Er lying on it.

Physician: Even ly:ing. Stan:ding up? walking aroun:d?
             ((singsong))

Patient: No: ⌈jis-⌉
Physician: ⌊Not⌋ so mu:ch. Jis'- ly:ing on it. Si:tting on it.
             Jis' then.

In this excerpt, the longest pause to ensue between the Black female
patient's response and the white male physician's next query is one
tenth of one second (marked by the period in parentheses). And, on
two occasions, the physician's "next" utterance cuts off the patient's
completion of her answer to his "last" one. The staccato pacing and
intrusions into the patient's turnspaces demonstrate that—in essence
and in fact—a simple "yes" or "no" is all this doctor will listen to. Such
practices also serve to demonstrate who is in control in this exchange.

In the case of both excerpts, it appears that the use of interruptions
by male doctors is a *display* of dominance or control to the patient,
just as males' and parents' interruptions (in my previous research)
were employed to communicate control in cross-sex and parent-child
exchanges. But also in these exchanges (as in the cross-sex and
parent-child data), I find that the use of interruptions is *in fact* a
control device, as the intrusions (especially when repeated) disorga-
nize the local construction of conversational activities. Insofar as the
over-arching conversational activity is, in the medical exchange, attending to the patient's health, we can only speculate on the potential
benefits being lost when doctors interrupt their patients.

Although Parsons tends to equate physicians' interactional control
over patients with the ability to treat them, I contend that this sort of
control is more likely to hinder than to help physicians' efforts at
healing. While it may be true, as he claimed, that patients consult

physicians because they do not know what is wrong with them nor what to do about it (Parsons, 1951:439), it is equally true that physicians must listen to patients in order to know what brings them there for treatment. Thus, the doctor—as well as the patient—has much to lose when one or the other of them is unable to "get a word in edgewise."

The Case of Female Physicians

The above analysis notwithstanding, the fact remains that results for four of the 21 exchanges in this collection do not display the asymmetrical pattern implied by Parsons's description. Exchanges between two women doctors and two women patients evidence distributions of interruptions that approach symmetry. Moreover, exchanges between female physicians and male patients show the male patients (not the female physicians) interrupting most (92 percent of interruptions in one exchange and 72 percent in another). It must be noted that there are only two female physicians interacting with two male patients in the collection of materials I analyze. Thus, attention to these dyads approximates a variant of case study rather than a survey of such participants generally. However, since these proportions parallel—rather than contradict—the actual distributions of females and males in medicine (where women, notes Judith Lorber, are "invisible professionals and ubiquitous patients," 1975), they would seem to warrant at least preliminary consideration here.

Permit me a brief digression to recall a somewhat dated riddle concerning a father and son who go for a ride in the country in the father's new sports car. Speeding too quickly around a corner, the father loses control of the wheel, and the car crashes into an embankment. The father is killed instantly, but the son is rushed to the local emergency room, where he is met by the hospital staff on call for emergency treatment. A surgeon rushes over to the stretcher, pulls back the blanket, and exclaims: "My God! I can't operate—that's my son!" The punchline of the riddle is: How can this be? If the boy's father was killed in the accident, then who is the surgeon?

The answer to the riddle—more obvious now, perhaps, than when it first came into vogue—is that the surgeon is the boy's *mother*. The usefulness of the riddle, as a heuristic device, rests in its illumination of the sorts of auxiliary traits that have come to accompany the status of "surgeon" in our culture. As Everett Hughes observes:

There tends to grow up about a status, in addition to its specifically determining traits [e.g., formal and technical competence], a complex of auxiliary characteristics which come to be expected of its incumbents. It seems entirely natural to Roman Catholics that all priests should be men, although piety seems more common among women. . . . Most doctors, engineers, lawyers, professors, managers, and supervisors in industrial plants are men, although no law requires that they be so. (1945:353–354)

In our society, notes Hughes, the auxiliary characteristics that have grown up around the status "physician" include "white," "Protestant," and "male." Therefore, when persons assume the powerful status of physician and are not possessed of whiteness, Protestantism, or maleness, there tends to be what Hughes terms a "status contradiction," or even a "status dilemma"—"for the individual concerned and for other people who have to deal with him" (1945:357).

The case of the "lady doctor" provides an illuminating example, the adjective "lady" (or "woman" or "female") only underscoring the presumed maleness of the status "physician."[6] Hughes argues that particular statuses (e.g., "Black") serve as "master-status determining traits," that is, traits which tend to have more salience than any others with which they may be combined. Thus, for persons (e.g., women) whose master-status conflicts with other very powerful statuses (e.g., physician), there is likely to be a dilemma over whether they are to be treated as members of the social category "women" *or* as practitioners of the profession "physician." Most important, as noted above, dilemmas of status extend not only to the individuals possessed of conflicting status-determining characteristics, but to those who must "deal with" them as well.

In the context of this analysis, we are well-advised to remember Zimmerman's (1978) observation that the appropriate behaviors of persons occupying social roles remain to be acted out in everyday life. Hughes's (1945) description might lead us to an overly deterministic perspective that portrays "choices" between two conflicting status-determining characteristics (e.g., "woman" and "physician"), as if the resolution of status dilemmas were an individual matter. However, the issue is more complicated than can be described by the "choice" or "nonchoice" of individuals who are caught in status dilemmas, since they must interact with others in their social worlds. For example, the Black man who would "pass" as a white one must rely on others' willingness to read various physical characteristics and elements of demeanor as constitutive of his "whiteness." Similarly, the woman who would become a physician must rely on others' willingness to honor her displays of professionalism over those of her gender.

While the evidence is tentative, there is reason to believe that Hughes's (1945) and Zimmerman's (1978) analyses might be pertinent to findings here presented. Recall, for example, that the four female physicians included in these exchanges were among the first cohort of women ever to enter the residency program at the Center. Moreover, at the time they began their training, there was only one woman physician on the staff of the faculty at the Center. (At the time of this writing, there is still only one faculty member who might ease the special adjustments of this "new and peculiar" cohort, through what might be termed role modeling, mentoring, or special advising, Shapiro et al., 1978.) Even the faculty supervising residents displayed a heightened awareness of the "special" status of the first cohort of women. For example, those who assisted me in my data collection took great pains to include "our new women residents" in the final corpus of exchanges.[7] Through such descriptions they helped make gender a salient characteristic for women residents (e.g., not once did I hear a doctor who was male described as a "man resident").

More pertinent still, for purposes of this data analysis, are the words of patients themselves. Consider the fragment below, excerpted from the final moments of one (white) female physician's first meeting with a new (Black female) patient:

(Dyad 11:740–747)

Physician: OKa:y!
                 (.6)
   Patient: °O:kay.
                 (.6)
Physician: We:ll, I've enjo:yed mee:ting you! hh
                 (.2)
   Patient: I ha:ve too::. Enjoy:ed meeting you:, cuz I've
              nev- .hh (.6) Nev:uh ha:d a fe:male docktuh
              befoah!-hunh-hungh-hungh-hungh!

"Enjoyable" or otherwise, meetings with female physicians are apparently rare in this patient's experience.[8]

Another (Black male) patient, asked by his (white) female physician if he was having any problems passing urine, responded "You know, the <u>doctor</u> asked me that" (transcribing conventions simplified here). In this instance, it was difficult to tell who "the doctor" *was*; "the doctor" was *not*, evidently, the female physician who was treating him.

Finally, consider the excerpt below, in which a (white) female physician attempts to provide her professional opinion on a (Black male) patient's problem:

(Dyad 4:213–231)

((To this point, the patient has complained about his weight, and the doctor and patient have been discussing possible strategies for reducing. One suggestion offered by the physician was to slow down while eating; but the patient has *just countered* that suggestion with a complaint—he does not like cold food.))

Patient: . . . An' they take twe:nny 'r thirdy minutes

.

. ((five lines deleted))

.

Tuh eat.
Physician: Wull what chew ⎡could DO: ⎤
Patient: ⎣An' then by the⎦ time they
         get through: their foo:d is col::d an' uh-
         'ey li:kes it y'know
Physician: ⎡engh-hengh-hengh-hengh-hengh⎤ .hh
Patient: ⎣An' th' they enjoy that   ⎦   but I- I
         'on't <u>like</u> cole foo:d.
                     (.2)
Physician: One thing yuh could <u>d</u> ⎡o::   ⎤
Patient: ⎣Spesh'ly⎦ food thet's
         not suhpoze: be <u>col</u>' =
Physician: = O:kay .h = is tuh ea:t, say,
         the <u>meat</u> firs'. Yuh know:, but if yuh have a
         <u>sal</u>:ad tuh eat, t' sa:ve that till <u>after</u> yuh eat
         the meat. (.) Cuz the <u>sal</u>:ad's <u>suh</u>pose tuh be
         co:ld.

Note that the physician's attempts to advance her solution are interrupted repeatedly by the patient's ongoing elaboration of his (already evident) problem.

In this same exchange, the patient earlier questioned his physician about a medication he is taking for high blood pressure. He said that he had heard a radio report indicating that this medicine "might" cause cancer. It was a controversial report since a great many people take that particular drug to help control their blood pressure elevations. The patient's concern is certainly one with which many of us can identify and it is especially poignant in these times (in which everything from saccharin to fluorescent lighting has been linked to some potentially serious health hazard). In the case of the patient's medication, the radio report was followed by a subsequent announcement advising people to continue taking their medicine since the research had confirmed no cause-and-effect relationship between the medication and cancer. The patient said that he never heard anything further (following the subsequent announcement).

Following this initial expression of concern, the doctor checked the patient's blood pressure and explained to him that she has looked into this problem. There is, she said, no alternative medication available, and there is, in her opinion, no better present alternative than to continue with his medication. At this juncture, the patient shifts to a slightly different complaint:

(Dyad 4:430–454)

Patient: . . . If there wuz any way <u>possible</u> duh git me
some diffrun' type a pill thet li:ke yuh take
twi:ce a da::y instead of three:, .hh an' have
th' same effeck with this (allernate) 'n u:h-
<u>wah</u>dur pi:ll,

Physician: OhKa:y, that's egzackly what we: were try:ing
tuh do:: .hh =

Patient: = Ah kno:w, but tho:se-
I- (.) heard ⎡what ⎤ th' man sai:d.

Physician: ⎣We:ll,⎦
               (.)

Physician: Ay:::e- checked <u>in</u>:ta tha:t, oka::y? an:::d-
(1.0) No:t No:t- <u>ex</u>tensively, I didn' search
all the lidda'chure =

Patient: = ((clears his throat))
      (.4)

Physician: .h Bu::t uh:m (.6) ((sniff)) Ah feel <u>comf</u>'trable
            us:in' thuh dru:::g? An' would take it muhself:::
            °If I needed tuh. ((Looking directly at the patient))
                                (6.0)
Physician: So it ⎡'s u:p- .hh It's u:p tuh you::   ⎤   ::=
Patient: ⎣But if all they sa:y- if there's any-⎦   =Ah
            know::w, it's u:h-uh ⎡bud it's u:h- ⎤ Ah'm try:in'
Physician: ⎣It's up tuh you:⎦
Patient: to: uh- .h ((clears throat)) i:s there: <u>any</u> <u>other</u>
            ty::<u>pe</u> that chew could u:h fi:gger . . .

To spare us, I have omitted the next several lines, in which the physician again asserts that there is nothing else the patient can take and
in which the patient again asserts his desire to get around taking this
medication. Below, however, is the resolution of their argument:

(Dyad 4:471–479)

Physician: <u>If I</u> brought cha some <u>ar</u>duhcul(s) saying thet
            this wuz Ok<u>ay</u>:::, would juh bih<u>lie</u>:::ve me? .h
Patient: Ye:ah, su:re, defin ⎡at'ly. ⎤
Physician: ⎣Oka:y.⎦
                                (.)
Physician: O ⎡Kay:,   ⎤ o::kay=
Patient: ⎣But u:h-⎦   =((clears throat)) .h Whether
            I would cha:nge to it'r no:t, it would be a diff-
            y'know, a nuther thi::ng,

The patient might "believe" this woman physician if she brought him
some articles supporting her opinions, but whether or not he would
follow her advice "would be a nuther thi::ng."

My concern here is not the possible carcinogenic effects of the drug
(though important)—nor the alternatives to it. Rather, I am interested
in the way in which this woman physician is "heard" by her (male)
patient (for further analysis of this excerpt, see Chapter 6). As noted
earlier, Parsons claimed that the therapeutic practice of medicine is
predicated on institutionalized asymmetry between physician and patient. In his view, physicians are in a position of situational authority
vis-à-vis their patients, since only physicians are possessed of the tech-

nical qualifications (and institutional certification) to provide medical care.

Yet, in these excerpts we see that neither technical qualifications (conferred by the training and medical degree) nor personal assurances ("I would take this myself," "I checked into it") are sufficient for the woman physician to have her authority (*as a physician*) respected by the patient. Elsewhere, Hughes (1958) suggests that clients of professionals do not simply grant them authority and autonomy as faits accompli. Given a recent history of increasing challenges to medical authority in the United States (cf. Reeder, 1972), it is entirely possible that patients in general are taking increased initiative in their own health care and questioning physicians' opinions more frequently. But nowhere in these data did I find a patient who questioned the opinion of a male physician as forcefully or as repeatedly as the case noted here.

Summary and Conclusions

Employing the model of turn-taking in conversation of Sacks et al. (1974), I established a theoretical basis for distinguishing interruptions from other types of simultaneous speech events in an attempt to examine the empirical bases for such claims as Parsons's (1951; 1975) regarding the essential asymmetry of the physician-patient relationship.

Exchanges between patients and male physicians in this collection lend support to the asymmetrical archetype: Male doctors interrupt their patients far more often than the reverse, and they appear to use interruptions as devices for exercising control in their interactions with patients. However, there is no evidence to suggest that this pattern of physician-initiated interruption is conducive to patients' good health. If anything, it appears that this sort of control is likely to hinder physicians' efforts at healing. Moreover, where female physicians are involved the asymmetrical relationship is exactly reversed: Patients interrupt their female doctors as much or more in each exchange in this collection. Thus, my results for women physicians conflict with Parsons's description of the general pattern.

At present, any discussion of the implications of this gender-associated difference must be speculative.[9] The corpus of materials does not constitute a random sample, and simple projections from these results to physicians and patients in general cannot be justified by the usual logic of statistical inference. But, in engaging in such discussion, I would hope to eliminate possible misinterpretations of its significance. I am not claiming that female physicians are "better listeners" than their male colleagues (although they may be).[10] These analyses have focused on the distribution of interruptions *between* physicians and patients. Whereas female physicians in this collection were interrupted by patients far more often than vice versa, it makes as much sense to attribute this finding to their patients' gender-associated "disrespect" (particularly in light of Hughes's and Zimmerman's suggestions) as it does to attribute it to the physicians' own communication skills. Neither inference is entirely warranted at this point.

What *is* tenable, for the findings reported here, is the suggestion that gender may have primacy over professional status where women physicians are concerned, that gender may amount to a "master–status" (Hughes, 1945), even where other power relations are involved.

CHAPTER 5

Questions and Answers Between Doctors and Patients*

Recently the television news magazine *Sixty Minutes* featured a story about a number of adults who had developed cancer in their lymph nodes following radiation treatments in early childhood. A mother who was interviewed on the program said that her (now adult) child had been given extensive X-ray treatments early in his life for what was described by the family physician as a "funny sounding" cry. When she was pressed by the *Sixty Minutes* interviewer to explain why she had allowed her child to undergo heavy doses of radiation for a relatively minor matter, the mother protested, "You never questioned a doctor in those days. The pediatrician was God!"

"God," in other words, was somebody not to be questioned. Ordinarily, though, we regard questions and answers as important means of exchanging information between people. The talk that occurs between a physician and patient would seem to offer a particularly important opportunity for an exchange of information, for here its presence or absence can have life and death consequences. From a practical perspective, patients appear to be the best sources of information on certain medical questions; certainly, they are doctors' sole sources of information regarding their subjective experiences of health and illness. So, we can understand how physicians might be predisposed to questioning their patients.

---

*An earlier version of these ideas appeared as " 'Ask Me No Questions . . .' An Analysis of Queries and Replies in Physician-Patient Dialogues," pp. 75–106, in S. Fisher and A. Todd (eds.), *The Social Organization of Doctor-Patient Communication* (Washington, D.C.: Center for Applied Linguistics, 1983).

But patients, too, should be similarly predisposed. On the occasions of visits to their doctors, patients come to petition them for information regarding medical care—information only physicians can provide (cf. Parsons, 1951). Thus, there are also good practical reasons for patients to question their physicians.

Whereas such pragmatic considerations would seem to facilitate the flow of information between patients and physicians, a growing body of literature suggests that the information exchanged in medical encounters is not always organized as a two-way "swap." For example, Korsch et al.'s (1968) investigation found that mothers' questions to pediatricians are often ignored, given ambiguous responses, or met with a change of topic by doctors (see also Paget, 1983; Todd, 1983). Wallen et al.'s (1979) report indicates that less than one percent of total time spent in information exchange is devoted to physicians' explanations to patients. And Frankel's (in press) analysis suggests that the overwhelming majority of physician-initiated utterances consist of questions to patients. Patient-initiated talk, in contrast, tends to be composed of anything *but* questions. These results lead Frankel to conclude that the form of talk which occurs in physician-patient "interviews" is a great deal more constrained by utterance-type and speaker identity than in casual conversation.

Frankel's suggestion illuminates a number of important issues for the concerns of this chapter. An interview is, by definition, a prestructured state of talk, characterized by a relatively "fixed" order of turns, length of turns, and content of turns (Sacks et al., 1974). Thus, one might expect an interviewer and interviewee to be alternating speaking turns composed of questions and answers (p. 710). But conversation is characterized by variable turn order, turn size, and turn content, all of which must be determined on a turn-by-turn basis. Hence, conversational exchanges present fewer restrictions on the form and content of speakers' utterances. If medical exchanges are primarily interviews, and only secondarily conversations, it will be difficult to maintain an open, two-way flow of questions and answers within their confines. Yet, since conversation is a relatively unstructured form of talk, it may be difficult to restrict purely conversational medical encounters to the 15-minute appointment slots they are typically allotted in physicians' daily schedules.

Of course, both "interviews" and "conversations" are forms of speech exchange that can be arranged on a continuum of lesser to greater prespecification. Each can contain elements typical of the other. Hence, questions and answers can be observed in the most casual of conversations, and sociable greetings and farewells can form boundaries around what otherwise might look like an interrogation (see Chapter 7). The crucial distinction between these forms of talk is, as Frankel notes, the degree to which they constrain the use of alternative types of utterances by different speakers. For example, in sociable chitchat "There is no necessity for one party to remain a questioner and another an answerer" (Frankel, in press:6). However, in a medical "interview" we would anticipate an asymmetrical exchange of questions and answers between doctors and patients, with physicians initiating the questions and patients providing the responses to them.

In this chapter, I offer an explicit empirical comparison of the initiation of questions and answers between patients and family physicians. I analyze the organization of these speech events as well as their consequences for subsequent talk, in order to understand why patients might have difficulty posing questions to doctors—even when their queries have a direct bearing on their state of health. My results support Frankel's claim that patient-initiated questions are "dispreferred" in medical dialogues.[1] Structural evidence for this dispreference is apparent in the very organization of patients' questions and physicians' replies to them. Since queries and responses are my units of analysis here, I begin by considering the status of questions and answers in speech exchange generally.

QUESTIONS AND ANSWERS

Grounding the theoretical status of questions (as questions) is more difficult than it might appear. To be sure, dictionaries provide definitions which concur with common sense, for example, "An interrogative sentence calling for an answer; an inquiry" (*Funk and Wagnalls*, 1964:1034), or "A sentence in an interrogative form, addressed to someone in order to get information in reply" (*The Random House College Dictionary*, 1975:1083). But patently self-evident definitions are found elsewhere, as well: "Within much of linguistics . . . the single sentence, abstracted from actual occasions of its use, serves as the unit of analysis . . . the properties of questions are seen as the self-contained . . . linguistic products of an individual speaker, irrespective of the communication situation itself" (Frankel, in press:35, fn. 7). While analysts of written texts may find that interrogative sentences compose the building blocks of questions they encounter, researchers faced with actual speech events will be forced to acknowledge alternative units of analysis. People, put simply, do not speak in the ways prescribed by dictionaries. For example, dialogues between physicians and patients (as between most people) exhibit many interrogative sentences coupled with requisite answers:

(Dyad 10:152–154)

Physician: Duh yuh ha:ve any <u>nu:mb</u>ness 'r <u>ti:n</u>gling?
    Patient: This- ha::n' stays numb all a ti:me.

But such exchanges also exhibit interrogative items that do not properly qualify as sentences, and even these may evoke answers:

(Dyad 10:156–158)

Physician: Thuh who:le hand? 'R jis' <u>part</u> of it.
    Patient: Muh fingers, mos'ly.

In this excerpt, for instance, "Thuh who:le hand?" is made intelligible as a query in the context of the fragment just above (i.e., the doctor's question regarding numbness or tingling and the patient's answer concerning the hand that stays numb all the time). Unto itself, however, "The who:le hand?" is not a grammatically complete sentence. Thus, it seems that questions do not have to be formulated as interrogative sentences in order to produce answers from their recipients. In fact, Sacks et al. (1974) suggest that speakers' turns at talk may be constructed of possibly complete words, phrases, clauses, or sentences, depending on their context. Since a question is one utterance-type that may occupy a speaker's turn, Sacks et al.'s proposal contradicts the usual dictionary definition. In other words, a sentence need not be uttered for a question to be asked.

And, just as less than a sentence will suffice, so will more. For example, Goffman (1981b:43) observes that speakers may launch series of questions in order to bury a single item as an unobtrusive element in a larger sequence. The ensuing sequence may itself unfold as a whole, to which increasingly abbreviated responses serve as replies (Shuy, 1974, cited in Goffman, 1981b). Frankel notes a complementary phenomenon in the abbreviation of questions into smaller question particles within question-answer chains:[2]

A: Does anybody have tuberculosis?
B: No, not that I know of
A: Heart disease
B: No
A: Diabetes
B: No

(Frankel, in press:12–13)

It is worth noting that only the first item in this series is formed with an interrogative intonational pattern. But, *as parts of the larger sequence,* we have little difficulty seeing "Heart disease" and "Diabetes" as items that warrant answers. Although intonational criteria are sometimes used to distinguish questions from other utterance-types, these grounds for distinction are shaky ones at best (cf. Lakoff, 1975:7). For example, the medical dialogues in this collection contain questions intoned as assertions:

(Dyad 19:548–550)

Physician:　.h An' yih been ha:vin' some i:tchin' in yer throat =
　Patient:　= Uh:, Uh-hu:h

And, they include answers with the intonational contours of questions:

(Dyad 15:466–468)

Physician:　°anything like tha:t?
　　　　　　　　(.8)
　Patient:　.h They <u>constantly</u> make that (.) cli:cking (.) cra:cking
　　　　　　sou::n?

Thus, there appear to be no ironclad intonational rules for distinguishing questions from other utterance-types.

Whereas these conceptual problems with "questions" are discouraging enough to potential analysts, Schegloff and Sacks (1974) note that the case for "answers" is even more obscure. They contend, for example, that purely linguistic criteria (syntax, semantics, phonology, etc.) offer no absolute rules for establishing utterances as "answers" to questions. Given minor variations in some paralinguistic features, items such as "yeah," "uh-huh," and "yep," often used to answer questions, may also be employed to convey acknowledgment, agreement, or understanding of another's utterance (see also Jefferson, 1973). Moreover, some questions (e.g., "d'yuh know what?") obligate their recipients to provide subsequent questions (e.g., "No, what?") rather than statements in response to them.

These considerations pose obvious methodological difficulties, leading some researchers to abandon questions and answers as appropriate units of analysis: "Our basic model for talk perhaps ought not to be dialogic couplets and their chaining, but rather a sequence of response moves with each in the series carving out its own reference, and each incorporating a variable balance of function in regard to statement-reply properties" (Goffman, 1981b:54). Certainly, Goffman is correct in arguing that conversation is not composed of predetermined utterance-types. Questions, statements, and responses may all furnish reasonable building blocks in a form of talk characterized by variable turn order, turn size and turn content. But for the analyst of medical exchanges, "dialogic couplets and their chaining" are not so easily replaced by alternative analytical units. If physician-patient talk is in fact organized as alternating "questions" and "answers," some way must be found to identify these and to distinguish them from other utterance-types.

Schegloff and Sacks (1974) contend that such utterance-types as answers to questions (or replies to summonses, responses to roll calls, etc.) only achieve their status as answers through their placement following questions. Answers form the second parts of what Schegloff and Sacks term *adjacency pairs;* as such, answers' intelligibility are *conditionally relevant* on the initiation of questions in the first instance. In other words, given the occurrence of a question, or "first pair part," an answer, or "second pair part," is anticipated. And, given the occurrence of a first pair part, an "absent" second pair part is notable: "We would expect that a Q followed either by silence or by talk not formulated as 'an answer' would provide the relevance and grounds for repetition of the Q or some inference based on the absence of an answer" (Schegloff, 1972:77). Hence, "an answer" ought to occur in

the next turn following completion of "a question"; if it does not, it
may be regarded as "officially" absent.

To be sure, this model does not dictate the uniform immediacy of
answers after questions. For example, "side sequences" (Jefferson,
1972) and "insertion sequences" (Schegloff, 1972) may intervene between an initial question and its answer without affecting the relationship of conditional relevance between the two. So, requests for
clarification or repetition may sometimes occupy the turns ordinarily
reserved for answers to initial questions:

(Dyad 11:007–009)

Physician: . . . 'Bout one fi:fy over ninedy. $\begin{bmatrix} \text{Uh-} \\ \text{How} \end{bmatrix}$ in the
    Patient:
                    world could she 'ave gotten tha:t?
Physician: <u>Par</u>don me:?
                    (.2)
    Patient: How in the world could she 'ave gotten that?

Here, for example, the physician's "<u>Par</u>don me:?" subsumes his answer to the patient's question.

Occasionally, one finds insertion sequences which are greatly protracted, with reiterative work occupying several turn rounds:

(Dyad 09:457–476)

Physician: One-twenny-ei:ght over one-oh-six.

                            · ((three lines deleted))

    Patient: (°One-oh-eight?)
                    (.4)
Physician: Hu:m?
                    (.2)
    Patient: One-oh-eight?
                    (.6)
Physician: One-oh-si:x
                    (1.2)

Patient: °Ah (men') thuh to:p nummer.

(.6)

Physician: One twenny eight.

However, even within protracted sequences, the conditional relevance of an eventual answer on the initial question can be seen. Just above, we can observe that the physician's "One twenny eight" does finally serve to answer the patient's initial query, in spite of the layers of reiteration between the two utterances. Where an insertion or side sequence occurs, then, it is in the turn's space immediately following completion of the sequence that an answer to an initial question is expected.

Quasi Question-types

Before proceeding further, a word of caution is in order. Schegloff and Sacks's (1974) analysis furnishes a clear distinction between the first pair part and second pair part of an adjacency pair, based on the respective temporal position of each component. In the case of questions and answers, this distinction means that an answer must follow a question in time and sequential position. Goffman makes a complementary observation: "Although a question anticipates an answer, is designed to receive it, seems dependent on doing so, an answer seems even more dependent, making less sense alone than does the utterance that called it forth. Whatever answers do, they must do this with something already begun" (1981b:5). Thus, questions appear to be forward-looking things, whose objects come recognizably next in a sequence of events. Answers, in contrast, have a retrospective flavor, and their sense must be garnered from that which preceded them. Therefore, the conditional relevance of answers on questions is not entirely reciprocal. Although answers' intelligibility depends on questions having been asked, the reverse is not true.[3]

This fact prompts consideration of some items that may be used to construct insertion and side sequences (see also Chapter 6). For example, an interrogative question term such as "Hunh?" and "What?" may be used to initiate a repair or repetition of another party's prior speech object, and thus orients its recipient backward, not forward, in sequential time. Repairs may also be initiated by partially repeating components of prior trouble-source turns, and by combining

"Y'mean" with some candidate understanding (guess) of another's prior object (Schegloff et al., 1977).

There are two other classes of conditionally relevant question-types which are found routinely in doctor-patient talk (and, for that matter, in casual conversation). One class might be called "requests for confirmation of a prior item." Included in my use of this description are declarative utterance-types (such as assertions) which are coupled with "Y'know?" "Okay?" "Like . . .?" or "Right?" to parody inquiries. Rather than to actually require an "answer," this form appears to provide an opportunity for the other to confirm or disconfirm some aspect of that to which it is appended.

Another class of conditionally relevant question-types consists of objects elsewhere identified (Schegloff, 1981) as markers of surprise, for example, "Really?" "Oh Really?" "Izzat so?" Even where responses to surprise markers occur, they too appear to be oriented to prior objects in a sequence.

In spite of variations in their form, then, all these devices share the retrospective quality of a search back to prior items in a sequence, and thus differ from other "questions" that might be asked.

In the analyses reported in this chapter, I do not include conditionally relevant question-types (requests for repair of prior items, requests for confirmation of prior items, and markers of surprise at prior items) in the general category of "questions" which call for answers. Since these objects look backward rather than forward in sequential time, they appear to be dependent for their sense on some equivalent of first pair parts.[4] Further theoretical grounds for separating such items from the general class can be found in consideration of their "answers." For example, when a request for repair is initiated in the turn following a question, the repair itself is a reiteration of the initial question:

(Dyad 8:308–315)

Patient: YUH GONNA DO THAT WITH MUH- MY
HU:RNEE TOO? ((the patient has perhaps had a hernia))

(1.0)

Physician: PARdun?

(.2)

Patient: YUH WAH- YUH WANNA SEE MY
             HURNEE ⎡TOO?⎤
Physician: ⎣Ye   ⎦ ah,

In this instance, for example, failure to separate the patient's repair from his initial formulation would result in a tally that counted the same question twice. Similar results would follow requests for confirmation of a question—the initial question, if confirmed, would be tallied doubly.

An independent analysis of the distribution of conditionally relevant question-types is, of course, of interest (and readers will find it in Chapter 6). However, it is important to distinguish such an analysis from the primary purpose of this chapter, the empirical description of the organization of questions and answers in medical dialogues. Interviews, for example, are not constructed out of alternating requests and repairs, but of alternating "questions" and "answers" (Sacks et al., 1974). As we now have a theoretically grounded basis for identifying these events, I turn next to present my findings.

Ask Me No Questions

Analysis began by examining the overall distribution of questions between the patients and Family Physicians in this collection. With the exception of conditionally relevant question-types, all possibly complete questions and answers (including nonverbal responses) were included for analysis, regardless of their content.[5] In the 21 exchanges and 532 pages of transcript, a total of 773 questions were observed (see Table 3). Of these, 91 percent (705) were initiated by doctors; 9 percent (68) were initiated by patients. In every dyad, doctors asked as many or more questions than did patients, and in 14 of the 21 exchanges, physicians initiated over 90 percent of the total questions asked.

Total numbers of questions display a broad range, with doctors asking as few as four and as many as 84 questions (in comparison to patients' range of zero to 18 questions asked). However, any clear trends toward symmetry with respect to age, sex, or race remain to be established.[6] One possible avenue for further investigation is illuminated by the especially asymmetrical exchanges between physicians and adolescent patients. Where teenagers were involved, we see that

TABLE 3

Questions in Encounters between
Physicians and Patients[1]

	Percentage of Physician-Initiated Questions		Percentage of Patient-Initiated Questions	
White male patient, 16 years	100	(41)	—	(0)
White female patient, 17 years	100	(41)	—	(0)
Black female patient, 16 years	100	(38)	—	(0)
White male patient, 16 years	100	(37)	—	(0)
Black female patient, 31 years	98	(54)	2	(1)
Black male patient, 36 years	97	(37)	3	(1)
White male patient, 38 years[2]	95	(19)	5	(1)
White female patient, 82 years	95	(84)	5	(4)
White female patient, 36 years	94	(15)	6	(1)
White female patient, 32 years	94	(31)	6	(2)
Black female patient, 67 years[2]	94	(45)	6	(3)
Black male patient, 17 years	94	(64)	6	(4)
White female patient, 58 years	92	(44)	8	(4)
White male patient, 36 years	91	(21)	9	(2)
Black female patient, 52 years[2]	89	(49)	11	(6)
Black male patient, 26 years	83	(15)	17	(3)
White male patient, 56 yeas	82	(23)	18	(5)
Black male patient, 58 years[2]	72	(18)	28	(7)
White male patient, 31 years	70	(7)	30	(3)
Black female patient, 20 years	57	(4)	43	(3)
White female patient, 53 years	50	(18)	50	(18)
Total	91	(705)	9	(68)

1. Dyads are hierarchically arrayed in order of increasing symmetry between physician and patient.
2. This patient visited a female physician; others visited males.

physicians asked 100 percent of the total questions in four cases out of five.[7] At the other end of the age continuum, a pattern is not so marked. The most symmetrical distribution of questions appears in an exchange between a physician and 53-year-old white female patient (in this dyad, each asked an equal number of questions). However, the next most symmetrical exchange occurred between a physician and a Black female patient who was 20 years of age. Thus, a clear trend toward increased symmetry of questions with greater patient age is not apparent.

What is apparent throughout these data is support for Frankel's (in press) claim that patient-initiated questions are "dispreferred" in doctor-patient dialogues (see Note 1, this chapter). Overall (and overwhelmingly), doctors ask the questions.

To be sure, interviews are constructed not only of questions, but of questions and answers in alternating turns at talk. The principles of adjacency pairs' organization dictate that answers should follow questions in time and sequential position. In these data, 96 percent of the total 773 questions asked (or 748) elicited answers from their recipients. However, the proportion of questions answered by patients and the proportion of questions answered by physicians is not equal. Of the 705 questions physicians asked, patients answered 98 percent (689). Of the fewer (68) questions patients asked, physicians answered 87 percent (59). Thus, while questions did, in the vast majority of cases, elicit answers from their recipients, patients answered physicians' questions more often than physicians answered theirs.

Doctors' Questions

Patients' "missing answers" often were noted in the vicinity of constraining structural circumstances. For example, where doctors chained a series of questions together with no intervening slots for answers, the individual queries that composed the chains frequently failed to elicit patients' responses:

(Dyad 5:358–363)

```
Physician:  NO: chi::lls? shakin' chi::lls?
   Patient:                                  ⎛Don'-⎞
Physician:                              =    ⎜high ⎟ fever? =
   Patient:  No:, jis- (.) slee:ping (.) alo:t (.) too:
   Patient:  ⎛That-⎞
Physician:  ⎝O    ⎠ kay.
```

Thus, in the above excerpt, if "chi::lls?", "shakin' chi::lls?", and "high fever?" are actually three separate queries, it is not clear to which (if any) of them the patient attempts a reply. (No nods or shakes of the patient's head were observed here.)

Further constraints on patients' answers were constructed through physicians' frequent utilization of "multiple-choice" questions. As in the case of their use in standardized tests, these queries may call for a bit more than "yes" or "no." But the very design of the questions leaves little doubt about how much more is permissible. Consider, for example, the extended series of queries posed in Dyad 10 (excerpted earlier):

(Dyad 10:152–162)

Physician: Duh yuh ha:ve any <u>nu:mbness</u> 'r <u>ti:ngling</u>?
            (1.0)
  Patient: This- ha::n' stays numb all a ti:me.
            (.2)
Physician: Thuh <u>who:le</u> hand? 'R jis' <u>part</u> of it.
            (.2)
  Patient: Muh fingers, mos'ly.
            (.2)
Physician: <u>A:ll</u> the fingers? 'R jis' <u>some</u> of 'em.
            (1.2)
  Patient: Yuh kno:w (1.4) when ah wuz in in the hospital . . .

Here, a sequence of "either/or" responses are embedded within the doctor's question construction (i.e., "<u>nu:mbness</u> 'r <u>ti:ngling</u>?", "Thuh <u>who:le</u> hand? 'R jis' <u>part</u>?", and "<u>A:ll</u> the fingers? 'R jis' <u>some</u>?"). More-over, the slots in which the patient's answers to individual queries could come (and should come, given the organization of adjacency pairs) are already occupied by the doctor's latching of forced-choice alternatives. In this way, the physician limits both the placement and content of possible patient replies.

Finally, as noted in Chapter 4, I found that where doctors' "next" questions were posed over patients' attempted answers to their "last" questions, incomplete answers often appeared within states of simul-taneous speech. Of the 16 physician-initiated questions which did not elicit answers from patients, 11 of them were positioned in chains or states of simultaneity in such fashion as to preclude slots for patient answers. Thus, patients' "failures" were very much products of the ways in which doctors posed their questions.

Patients' Questions
As we have seen, patient-initiated queries were relatively rare oc-currences in these exchanges, comprising only 9 percent of the total

questions asked. In fact, only one of the 21 encounters contained more than ten patient-initiated questions, and that dyad exhibited more symmetry in the distribution of questions between physician and patient than any other in this collection. Given their scarcity, it is notable that patient-initiated questions failed to elicit answers from physicians more often than the reverse (13 versus 2 percent respectively). Still more notable is the fact that the greatest number of physician failures were observed in the exchange in which the patient asked most questions. A total of nine questions were not answered by doctors; of these, four were initiated by the patient in this single exchange. Thus, a detailed examination of this exchange may shed some light on the circumstances under which patients' questions are ignored, given ambiguous responses or met with a change of topic by doctors (cf. Korsch et al., 1968).

An indirect precursor to one question in this exchange is not completed by the patient:

(Dyad 1:615–626)

    Patient: When Tack-o-cardia star::ts, have you god any goo:d
                sugges- like jus' now:, I- I suddenly felt sort of
                a .hh- hh (.2) thing starting in my throat, which is of
                'un a
                                        (.2)   (work for)
    Physician: Uh- does the (Mac Craw::: sa:w- massage (do anything
                for) yuh sometimes? ((stroking his throat))
                                        (.)
    Patient: Sometimes

In this instance, the patient's initial query is dropped midway into the utterance, and left hanging incomplete. But it has evidently been recognized by the physician, who offers a counter-question as a candidate "good suggestion" (albeit, one that works only "sometimes" for the patient). A side sequence follows, leaving further completion and elaboration of the initial query unfinished by the patient.

However, shortly thereafter we find the first "official absence" of an answer to a possibly complete question:

(Dyad 1:634–640)

> Patient: .h Well, I've been taking Did-jox-cin three times a day,
> though I understand juh can take it all <u>on::ce</u>, if you
> wan'. Is- izat ri::ght? =
>
> Physician: = You've been taking point-one-two-five three times a
> day ev'ry day:, °right?
>
> (.)
>
> Patient: °Ye:ah. =
>
> Physician: = °O:kay ((makes a note))
>
> (1.0)

Again, an insertion sequence intervenes just after the initial query, leaving it unanswered. Once this sequence is completed, though, the patient begins reformulating her prior incomplete question:

(Dyad 1:649–657)

> Patient: Ye:ah. Uh- fou::r times a day fer tha:t, an'
> La:n-ox-cin I been taking three:: times a day. <u>So.</u>
> If I <u>start</u> into a:: (.) ((leans back in the chair
> again)) into a- uh- ah: Pa- Pee Ay Tee:
>
> (.8)
>
> Physician: How: long 'ave you been takin' that- three times a day.
>
> (1.0)
>
> Physician: A long time?
>
> (.)
>
> Patient: Ye:ah. ((nodding))

Once more, the question is left hanging, supplanted by a physician-initiated insertion. And in the concluding stages of this sequence, the patient reiterates her earlier completed but still unanswered query:

(Dyad 1:671–682)

> Physician: thet's high- <u>hi:gh</u>er thun the u:sual <u>dose</u>.
> (.) Fer a woman of yer si:ze.
>
> (.)

Patient: °Mm. Wull- he 'ad <u>to:le</u> me I could take all <u>three:</u>
of thum at <u>on::ce.</u>

(.)

Physician: Ye:ah, yuh ca::n.
Patient: An' I thoud it'd be bedder duh space it ou:t 'n- it rilly
doesn make any diff'runce?

(.2)

Physician: It- we::ll hh-hh Taking <u>tha:t</u> dose, ((pointing with
his pen to the sheet in front of him)) I'd- I'd
I'd rather see yuh space 'em ou:t.

Thus, a "straight answer" to this question is still notably absent. The
physician has not confirmed that "it really doesn't make any difference"; on the other hand, he has not indicated that it does. Instead,
he offers his preference for what she ought to do ("I'd rather see yuh
space 'em out"), minus an explanation.

In the wake of this failure, another problematic sequence occurs:

(Dyad 1:684–720)

Patient: Um-hmm:.
Physician: Now: if = ⎡'e = wuz = taking-⎤
Patient: ⎣Wull isn' it   ⎦ on my <u>re:cord?</u>
((she brings her hand down on the desk,
index finger first, as if pointing)) when 'e had
the le:vels measured? ((pulls her hand back now))
it <u>shou::ld</u> be:

(1.0)

Physician: ((flipping back through the pages in her file))
Le:mme check.

·

·

· ((13 lines deleted))

Physician: [No::] [I <u>don't</u>] see a dih-jox-cin level here anywhere.

(.6)

Patient: Wull he's had that taken, at <u>least</u> <u>twi::ce,</u> that I
rihmember.

·

·

· ((two lines deleted))

Physician: ((still rifling through her file)) Uh-hunh::
                                    (2.4)
Physician: Wuzzat in a <u>hos</u>pidul? you had it taken? ((still rifling))
                                    (.2)
   Patient: <u>He</u>:::re. ((points over her shoulder to the door behind
           her))
                                    (1.0)
   Patient: At this cli:nic. ((brings her hand down again))
Physician: Hmm::m, °Okay. ((still lifting page after page))
                                    (6.8)
Physician: Hm-um-um-umph! ((yawning)) 'Scu:se me, mm:
                                    (12.0)
Physician: We:ll. ((puts file aside and looks up)) I'd like tuh
           measure that tuhda:y an' see whuddit i:s, cuz I-
           like I sa:y, id i:::s (.) a higher than average dose.

The question at issue here ("Wull isn' it on my <u>re:cord</u>?") is remark-
able on a number of counts. It is formulated as a direct question
(rather than as a "tag," for example), it interrupts the doctor's utterance (see Chapter 4), and it constitutes a challenge by the patient
regarding the manner in which her records have been kept at the
Center. Further, when the physician fails to provide a direct response
("I <u>don't</u> see a dih-jox-cin here"), the patient elaborates her query
("<u>Wull</u> he's had that taken, at <u>least</u> twi::ce"). Even at this, following a
considerable delay and numerous gaps in talk, the doctor announces
that he will himself take another measurement—without ever having
provided a direct response to the patient's question.

   The patient's initially incomplete and indirect question (about her
excessively rapid heartbeat) does finally receive an answer from the
doctor, much later in this exchange:

(Dyad 1:749–760)

   Patient: .hh Alright. So if I fe- fee:l this coming on, an'
           I'm sidding up in a <u>pla:ne</u>, 'r I'm out somewhere in
           a <u>ca:r</u>, .h 'n I c ⎡an't lie dow-   ⎤
Physician: ⎣LIE:: DOW:N!⎦
   Patient: = Wull, spoze I can' lie <u>dow:n</u>
                                    (1.0)

Physician: 'F yuh can' ((tosses his head)) lie down, yih can'
lie dow:n. =

Patient: = °Mm =

Physician: = Uh::: si:t calmly, (.) an'
take a Valium.

(1.0)

Physician: An' the:n, I'd try thuh thro:at (craw-sage) massage
firs'. Jis' keep it gen'rally steady fer about
twenny-thirdy sekkins. 'F it doesn'- swi:tch within
that time, try: th' other one

Note, however, that eliciting an answer to this question has required three separate attempts by the patient. When the doctor's answer eventually emerges, it appears over one hundred lines later in the transcript than the patient's initial formulation of her query.

Repeatedly in these excerpts, we see patient-initiated questions subsumed and circumvented by physician-initiated activities (e.g., counter-questions to patient questions and consultation of the ever-available medical files). Circumvention necessitates considerable agility in this exchange, since the patient is far more articulate (by conventional standards) than many other patients. Her use of medical terminology is relatively sophisticated, she exhibits an active, sometimes challenging curiosity about the state of her health, and she consistently repeats her questions when they go unanswered. However, she evidences *more* difficulty in getting answers to her questions than any other patient in this collection. Though impossible to prove here, it is entirely likely that this patient's very assertiveness is associated with her difficulties. If physicians normatively ask the questions and patients normatively respond to them, a general dispreference for patient-initiated questions may be reflected in this doctor's reluctance to answer "too many" of them.

The Structural Deviance of Patient-Initiated Questions

Stronger evidence of the dispreferred status of patient questions is furnished by closer inspection of the forms they take. In the course of this analysis, I assembled a collection of all patient-initiated questions from these exchanges. What is most striking in this collection is the presence of marked speech perturbations in the speech objects used by patients to construct their queries. For example, even in the dyad just inspected, the onset of patient questions was routinely marked by hitches or stutters in the patient's production of an object:

(Dyad 1:634)

Patient: I understand juh can take it all on::ce,
if you wan'. Is- Izzat ri::ght?

(Dyad 1:649)

Patient: If I start into a::: (.) into a- uh- ah:
Pa- Pee Ay Tee:

(Dyad 1:749)

Patient: So if I fe- fee:l this coming on,

Similar disfluencies are evident in other excerpts presented earlier:

(Dyad 8:035)

Patient: Can YOU TELL- HOW SOMEBODY CUN EAT- EAT
U:H- WHAT CHA EAT- EAT IN THE BLOOD?

In fact, of the total of 68 questions posed by patients, 46 percent (31) displayed some form of speech disturbance in the course of their production. Put simply, patients displayed considerable difficulty "spitting out" their questions.

But their difficulties exhibited no systematic patterns. In a few cases, stutters and hitches appeared in questions that might have been associated with patients' anxieties:

(Dyad 18:299)

Patient: Ah me:an, i::s it ri:ll serious? Iz- izzit
somethin' that could-

(Dyad 7:993)

Patient: Wull that- Is that nor:mul? I mean is tha:t oka::y?

Certainly, a body of literature evolving from speech therapists' studies links stuttering in general to topics that are anxiety-producing for

speakers. But in these exchanges, stutters also appear in questions
about matters of relatively little consequence to patients:

(Dyad 6:051)

    Patient: Wu- yuh can' take the thing ((a scab on his finger))
           off tuhda:y?

(Dyad 9:514)

    Patient: Ah nodice' peepul put salt all ovuh theah body when
           they wuh in thuh steam bath. S- Whut's that foah?
           duh yuh kno:w?

In some instances, stutters appeared in close proximity to what
Schegloff et al. (1977) term "self-repairs." One may initiate repairs of
one's own utterance by dropping objects midway through production
in order to substitute alternative formulations for them:

(Dyad 2:232)

    Patient: Was my blood pr- Wha' wuz my blood pressure this
           ti:me?

Just above, for example, a possible question + assessment (i.e., "Was
my blood pressure high?", "Was my blood pressure low?", "Was my
blood pressure okay?") is replaced with a request for the information
on which an assessment might be based. In another instance in which
reformulation occurred, a patient's own assessment is retracted for a
soliciting of the physician's opinion:

(Dyad 4:002)

    Patient: Ah had a couple of uh: nose: bleeds an': Ah guess
           meybe that's (1.0) .h whadduh yuh think that:t come
           from

Some patient stutters preceded self-corrections of apparent errors
in objects under production:

(Dyad 14:712)

    Patient: Wull is iss a:ll due for- from th' hear::t?

(Dyad 8:308)

> Patient: YUH GONNAD DO THAT WITH MUH- MY
> HUR:NEE TOO?

But others preceded replacements of speech objects with those same objects just suspended by the stutters:

(Dyad 11:595)

> Patient: Whut would uh: keep- keep me from ha:vin' it flex?

(Dyad 1:736)

> Patient: Wh- when will yuh have the rihsul:ts (.2) the tes's
> you'll have taken tuhda:y, tuhmor:row?

Hence, the items which followed stutters did not necessarily "correct" anything.

In some cases, possibly "presumptive" queries were downgraded to less forceful forms:

(Dyad 18:372)

> Patient: Won' I- (.4) Wull I be gettin' a hot- ho:t pad
> from it?

Elsewhere, the objects that followed hitches appeared to be stronger formulations than those which preceded them:

(Dyad 4:454)

> Patient: Ah'm try:in' to: uh- .h ((clears throat))
> i:s there: any other type: that chew could
> u:h fi:gger aroun:' it?

Whether they were upgraded, downgraded, or regraded with the same material, patients' reformulations all displayed the troublesomeness of asking doctors questions.[8]

In all the exchanges containing patient-initiated questions (17 of the total 21), only one (white female) patient managed to produce her single question without a hitch:

(Dyad 5:161)

Patient: Yeah:, y' get those 't drugstores?

In the case of every other patient (female and male, Black and white) who asked questions in these exchanges, some (if not all) questions were marked by stuttering.

One should not interpret these results to mean that a singularly inarticulate group of patients was included in this data base. To the contrary, even relatively articulate patients (e.g., the white female in Dyad 1), whose speech was quite fluent in other contexts, displayed noticeable disturbances when asking questions of doctors. What these findings do suggest is that patients also treat self-initiated questions as somehow problematic.

NORMATIVE STRUCTURES OF PHYSICIAN-PATIENT DISCOURSE

I began this chapter with an anecdote, illustrating the lofty heights inhabited by entities "not to be questioned." Recall that from one patient's vantage point, both God and the family physician had achieved such exalted status. On the basis of results reported here, I would have to conclude that some physicians indeed inhabit a privileged position (if not a state of grace) with respect to being questioned by their patients.

As we have seen, patients initiated only 9 percent of the 773 questions posed in these exchanges. Some patients were involved in exchanges with physicians they had known for three years at the time of recording; others were meeting physicians for the first time. Some visits were prompted by long-standing problems, while others were impelled by discoveries of new complaints. Despite these variations, medical exchanges exhibited a systematic and asymmetric pattern: Overwhelmingly, physicians asked the questions. The consistency of this pattern offers considerable support for Frankel's notion that patient-initiated questions are dispreferred in physician-patient dialogues.

These findings further suggest that medical exchanges are more constrained by utterance-type and speaker identities than casual conversation, consistent with Frankel's claims to this effect. Not only do doctors ask the questions in this collection of exchanges, but patients provide the responses to them. Hence, as we saw earlier, patients answered 98 percent of the questions asked by doctors. But doctors, who were asked far fewer questions by their patients, also responded to fewer of those they were asked.

Assuredly, the majority of patients' questions *were* answered by physicians in this collection. Moreover, only five of the 21 exchanges exhibited physicians failing to answer patients' questions. Thus, it would be incorrect to conclude that patients' questions were generally ignored by physicians in these dyads. While the results of Korsch et al. (1968) showed patient questions frequently neglected, given vague answers, or countered by changes of subjects by physicians, my own results indicate most patient questions are answered. There are, of course, major differences in our methods of data collection. Korsch and her colleagues conducted their study in a large teaching hospital, while my investigation was done in a small clinic. Whereas their research design treated mothers as patients in pediatric exchanges, my analysis was confined to two-party interactions between adult patients and Family Physicians. Therefore, methodological differences preclude strict comparison of our findings.

Even so, our results exhibit some parallels. In Korsch et al.'s survey of 800 patient visits, "10% of mothers asked no questions and an additional 27% asked only one or two" (p. 864). In my collection of 21 exchanges, 19 percent of patients asked no questions of physicians, and 29 percent asked one or two. In other words, 48 percent of the exchanges (10 of the 21) contained two or fewer patient questions. Further, in the single dyad exhibiting a symmetrical distribution of questions between doctor and patient (also exhibiting the largest number of patient-initiated questions), I observed the largest number of physician failures to answer patient questions. This finding corresponds with results obtained by Wallen et al. (1979), who report that the patients who asked most questions were not necessarily the ones who received most explaining time (p. 145). Indeed, the dispreference for patient-initiated questions in this collection may be displayed by physicians' reluctance to answer "too many" of them (cf. Roter, 1977). In quantitative terms then, the scarcity of patients' questions and their lesser likelihood of being answered by physicians indicates that patient-initiated questions are not the preferred organizing devices for medical dialogues.[9]

Qualitative analysis suggests a similar conclusion. For example,

physicians exhibited a tendency to formulate some questions that limited patients' options for placement and content of responses. Where
doctors latched individual queries into chains, posed multiple-choice
questions, and initiated next questions over patients' answers to prior
queries, they reduced (or eliminated) patients' slots for answers. As
others have noted (e.g., Sacks, 1966; Ray and Webb, 1966; Shuy,
1976; Goffman, 1981b; Frankel, in press b), the use of utterance-
types containing multiple components can itself constrain opportunities for responses. Thus, both the numbers of doctors' questions and
the ways they are constructed exhibit an orientation to a normative
order of medical discourse in which physicians' question are
preferred.

Patients' questions also exhibit this orientation. As we have seen,
patients' infrequent questions to doctors were often marked by speech
disturbances. Though some stutters preceded questions that may
have been anxiety-provoking for patients, not all of them did. And
while some stutters preceded patient reformulations of questions,
other "reformulations" emerged as formulations of the same items
that were stuttered. So, while repairs and reiterations exhibited no
consistent patterns according to what, if anything, they "fixed," they
did provide considerable evidence of patients' difficulties "spitting
out" their questions. Through the very talk they produce, patients
seem to display a dispreference of self-initiated queries.

To be sure, many other activities are routinely in progress while
physicians and patients converse. More than a few of them may be
associated with the distribution of questions and answers reported
here. For example, diagnosis is often described as an activity concerned with hypothesis-testing, in which an ordered sequence of theories is subjected to an ordered set of proof procedures.[10] In this
view, physicians talking with patients are seen as simultaneously engaging in cognitive processing of information regarding their patients' states of health:

> When a physician first confronts a prospective patient, she (he) is uncer-
> tain of the patient's medical problems. Some indication of what is both-
> ering the patient may have been elicited at the time an appointment was
> made, or is elicited by a nurse . . . when the patient arrives. The doctor
> begins to hypothesize about possible alternatives almost immediately.
> Each hypothesis leads to one or more subroutines requiring information
> retrieval from the doctor's and the patient's memory. Question-answer

sequences evolve, changing their course and content sometimes abruptly. The physician must stimulate the patient's memory concerning relevant events prior to and after the onset of the problem. The physician obviously believes that the patient can help her if her questions are put properly. (Cicourel, 1981b:94)

Thus, since information processing is conducted in deductive fashion, a patient's question may be seen as constituting an interruption of the physician's deductive thought process (see also Cicourel, 1975; 1978; 1981a; Måseide, 1983). Of course, this perspective also views diagnosis primarily as a cognitive process (transpiring within the physician's head) rather than as an interactional one (evolving between doctor and patient in the course of their talk with one another). Some might argue that results of this investigation might be explained through consideration of similar activities external to doctor-patient talk. However, at this point in our knowledge, these "explanations" do not have the status of reasons, but of hypotheses, requiring further exploration.[11] Therefore, I would suggest that they might be more usefully employed as the bases for future studies than as explanations for results obtained in this one.

SUMMARY AND CONCLUSIONS

The implications of these findings also provide grounds for present speculation and future inquiries. We might, however, indulge in some preliminary consideration of their potential import, given the context of the physician-patient relationship in the larger society of which it is a part. First, we can note that the production of medical "interviews" (i.e., states of speech exchange in which doctors ask the questions and patients answer them) is a thoroughly interactional accomplishment. As we have seen, this order of affairs is not merely an outcome of patients' passivity nor of physicians' dominance. Rather, the dispreference we observed for patient-initiated questions is produced jointly by physicians and patients in the course of their talk with one another. Not only do doctors advance questions which restrict patients' options for answers, but patients themselves stammer when asking questions of their doctors. Both physicians and patients are implicated in this social construction of reality. Thus, as Frankel (forthcoming) observes, "it would be inappropriate to view the issues of control and responsibility in the medical encounter as properties of individuals"

(p. 33). Instead, we are compelled to view such matters as micropolitical achievements, produced in and through actual turns at talk.

Second, we might note that physicians' and patients' evident preference of doctor-initiated questions parallels the presumed roles of physicians and patients in the larger system of social action. Certainly it is no accident that the physician—that is, "the technical expert who by special training and experience, and by an institutionally validated status, is qualified to 'help' the patient" (Parsons, 1951:439)—is the one who asks the questions in these encounters. Given that questions initiate activities that restrict and mandate subsequent grounds for action by their recipients (Frankel, in press:5), physicians' positions in larger order structural arrangements dictate that they, rather than patients, will properly be the ones to invoke those restrictions and mandates.

Third, we might observe that large-scale institutional arrangements provide an additional rationale for patients' evident discomfort while asking doctors questions. For example, one patient, after politely but firmly pressing his doctor to explain his long-standing back problems, said "Ah'm not tryin' duh pla:y docktuh:. Cuz zat's not muh fie::l'." Within his denial, we see the tacit suggestion that asking questions is tantamount to playing doctor (and playing doctor may be tantamount to playing God.) Thus, while patients may indeed have practical and pressing concerns that predispose them to query physicians, the very premise on which their relationship is based may discourage patients from employing this means to solicit information from their doctors.

This chapter has utilized work in conversation analysis to develop a theoretical framework for analyzing the organization of questions and answers between patients and family physicians during routine visits to the doctor. My explicit comparison of the initiation of questions and answers finds an asymmetric distribution of utterance-types, in which patients provide responses and doctors ask the questions. Whether this is the best way or the only way for organizing medical encounters is a matter of heated personal opinion for many. But it is also a matter for continuing scholarly investigation. Only through systematic empirical study of the minutiae of medical exchanges can we learn what constitutes the alleged communication "gap" between doctors and patients, and how it might be transformed.

CHAPTER 6

Medical Misfires: Mishearings, Misgivings, and Misunderstandings*

> One patient thought that being on a low-salt diet was bad enough. Then, in the hospital, she discovered to her dismay that she was also put on a low-sodium diet. (Silver, 1979:4)

Whenever people venture to talk, they run the risk of not being heard or understood. In sociable chitchat, the consequences of "unhearings," mishearings, and misunderstandings are serious enough, involving potential embarrassment, offense to others, and discrediting of oneself (cf. Goffman, 1967:97–113; 1981b). But when instrumental activities are coupled with dialogic ones, both may be endangered by failures to establish mutual intelligibility between speakers. Hence, during lectures, lessons may be lost as the result of inattention to furrowed brows and raised ones (cf. Schegloff, 1981:2). In debates, contests may be ceded through failures to hear and rebut another's contentions. And, in medical encounters, lives may be lost in the wake of misunderstandings between physicians and patients.

For at least thirty years, studies have indicated that physician-patient dialogues are particularly vulnerable to mishearings and misunderstandings by participants (e.g., Redlich, 1945; Seligmann et al., 1957; Ley and Spelman, 1967; Boyle, 1970; Korsch and Negrete, 1972; McKinlay, 1975; and Silver, 1979).[1] Some investigators suggest that a major impediment to mutual intelligibility is posed by doctors'

---

*An earlier version of these ideas was titled "Medical misfires: Mishearings, misgivings and misunderstandings in physician-patient dialogues," *Discourse Processes* 7 (1984):107–134. Alliterative inspiration for the title comes from Grimshaw (1980).

and patients' failures to communicate in the same language. Thus, Ley and Spelman (1967) note that commonly used diagnostic terms may convey little—or erroneous—meaning to patients; Korsch and Negrete (1972) report that physicians' descriptions are often "Greek" to their patients; and McKinlay (1975) observes that though patients are more familiar with medical terminology than physicians think they are, they do not know very much (see also Shuy, 1976). "Retrospectively," one doctor remarks, "it is not surprising that patients do not understand much of what we tell them" (Silver, 1979:5).

Unfortunately (for clinical practice) much of our analytic understanding of medical miscomprehensions is also acquired retrospectively. For example, Korsch and Negrete learned that pediatricians' instructions were "Greek" to mothers by interviewing mothers *following* their visits to pediatricians. Ley and Spelman managed to pinpoint those medical terms that were confusing to patients by administering multiple choice examinations to them after initial interviews. Other investigators (e.g., Wallen et al., 1979) have employed retrospective questionnaires to assess doctors' and patients' attitudes toward encounters that have already transpired between them (see the review of these studies in Chapter 2 and an excellent overview by Ley, 1983). In short, physicians' and patients' misperceptions have only been identified in the aftermath of the dialogues in which they were produced.

While this research has been helpful in calling attention to the existence of problems of intelligibility between physician and patient, it is of limited practical use in developing solutions to the problems. For example, how are physicians to know, in the context of actual encounters with patients, which words might not be familiar to them? Further, how are patients to know, while talking with physicians, when they have been heard incorrectly? In real life situations doctors and patients have no way of assessing one another's reactions to words that they use *as they use them* other than by observing the other's responses to them at that time.

Certainly, within any form of talk, devices exist for ensuring intelligibility between speakers. One obvious means to this end is asking, that is, posing a direct question. However, where the use of questions is restricted, so too may opportunities be limited for identifying speakers' troubles. Here again, there are grounds for suspecting that physician-patient talk may be especially fraught with difficulties. As

we saw in Chapter 5, questions are not freely available to all participants in medical dialogues. Korsch et al. (1968) found mothers' questions were ignored or given vague responses by pediatricians; Wallen
et al. (1979) report that patients receive very little explaining time
from their doctors; Frankel (in press) observes that patients' questions
are dispreferred in medical exchanges; and my own analysis indicates
that doctors—not patients—ask the questions.

The pronounced asymmetries I found in the distribution of questions and answers between doctors and patients seemed to suggest
that the physician stands in nearly "godlike" status in relation to a
patient, as an entity "not to be questioned." Whatever their state of
grace, though, doctors also risk losing much when mishearings and
misunderstandings pass unnoticed. In medical dialogues, a lack of
mutual intelligibility may result in mis-diagnosis, mis-treatment, and
even charges of malpractice. Given these dangers, it seems reasonable
to explore the possibility that some alternative to direct questions
might be available to ensure that physicians and patients are heard
and understood by one another.

In this chapter, I extend the preceding analysis of questions and
answers in medical encounters to a further consideration of
"question-like" items that do not serve to elicit "answers" per se. Although these interrogative forms are frequently treated as residual to
the "real" work of information exchange,[2] they are in fact primary
means available to speakers for establishing ongoing hearing and understanding of talk itself. Included here, for analysis in their own
right, are requests for repair of prior utterances, such as, "What?"
(Schegloff et al., 1977); requests for confirmation of prior utterances,
for example, an assertion appended by "Yuh know?" (see Chapter 5);
and markers of surprise at prior utterances, such as, "Rilly?" (Schegloff, 1981). My analysis of the use of these devices indicates that
though patient-initiated questions may be strongly dispreferred in
doctor-patient exchanges, patient requests for confirmation, repair,
and markers of surprise are not. Moreover, the local contexts in which
these devices are employed indicate strategic points at which diagnosis and treatment regimens are jointly forged between physicians and
patients. In discussion of these results, I consider their possible implications for issues of patient satisfaction, the organization of medical
interviews, and the potential for achieving more symmetrical relations
between physicians and patients.

Recall that the preceding chapter employed Schegloff and Sacks's (1974) discussion to establish a theoretical basis for identifying questions and answers in medical dialogues. Organizationally, a question and answer constitute what Schegloff and Sacks term the "first pair part" and "second pair part" of an *adjacency pair,* that is, a two-part sequence of talk constructed by two different speakers in adjacent positions to one another. As the second pair part of a question-answer adjacency pair, an answer's intelligibility is seen to be conditionally relevant on a question having been asked. Thus, an "answer" is a retrospective device, whose status as an answer can only be derived from what has preceded it (Schegloff and Sacks, 1974). A "question," in contrast, is a forward-looking thing, whose object (a reply) comes recognizably next in a series of utterances (Goffman, 1981b:5).

So, given that a first pair part, such as a question, is initiated, a second pair part, such as an answer, is expected. And, if the expected "next" does not occur (e.g., a silence ensues), its absence is noticeable (Schegloff, 1972:77). The adjacency pair organization of questions and answers thus provides theoretical warrant for the expectation that answers will appear in the turnspaces following questions. Moreover, this organization permits us to notice the "official" absence of "answers" vis-à-vis specifiable structural criteria.

Such considerations prompt the analysis of those speech objects at issue here. For example, while classifying "questions" and "answers," I observed numerous queries that seemed to evoke reproductions of utterances that were produced in preceding turns. One type employed an interrogative question term to initiate a repetition or "repair" of an utterance just produced by another party to talk (Schegloff et al., 1977):[3]

(Dyad 9:408–412)

    Patient: Seem lahk ah (°lean since ah been comin' duh
               Fam'ly Pracdice.) hunh-°engh!
    Physician: What?=
    Patient: =.h Ah said ah've learn' a <u>lot</u> since ah been
               been comin' duh Fam'ly Pracdice.

In the fragment just above, the reply to "What?" is a restatement of the utterance just preceding it. Thus, "What?" orients its recipient backward, rather than forward, in sequential time. Other terms that can be used in this fashion are "Who?" "Hunh?" "Where?" "When?" (Schegloff et al., 1977) and the less colloquial "Pardon me?"[4]

Schegloff et al. note that repairs may also be requested by partially repeating another party's trouble-source turn:

(Dyad 2:198–201)

Physician: Any (°mo:ss) in yer (.2) bladder? 'r ⌈°bowel problum⌉ =
Patient: ⌊Mo:::ss?   ⌋
Patient: = Nuho, my bladder's fine =
Physician: = Uh-kay

And they may be initiated by appending "Y'mean . . ." to some candidate understanding (i.e., guess) of prior speech objects (Schegloff et al., 1977):

(Dyad 10:319–322)

Patient: An' ah cun take thi:s hand an' li:ft it, an' it duh'unt
         hurt.
Physician: Yuh mean, when yuh <u>lif</u> the ar:m up, using yer other
         han:d? =
Patient: = Uh-huh.

While their forms vary, all of these *requests for repair* exhibit the retrospective quality of a search back to prior items in a sequence.[5] Thus, as noted in Chapter 5, these objects differ markedly from "questions" per se: they look backward instead of forward in sequential positioning.

A second class of backward-looking items I have termed *requests for confirmation*.[6] These objects tie declarative utterances (such as assertions) with "Y'know?" "Okay?" and "Like . . .?" in simulated inquiries:

(Dyad 2:027–028)

Patient: It hur:::ts, ok ⌈ay:?   ⌉
Physician: ⌊°Mm-hmm⌋

For example, in this fragment (presented earlier), the physician's acknowledgment token overlaps the patient's queried "okay?" But the acknowledgment token cannot be seen as a legitimate "answer" to a "question," for what would the question be? Surely, the patient is not asking her doctor for "permission" to hurt, nor does it seem that she is seeking the physician's clinical assessment of her pain (e.g., "Is it okay if it hurts?" or "Is it still healing properly even if it causes pain?"). Rather, it appears that "okay?" offers an opportunity for the physician to confirm or disconfirm the intelligibility of the utterance so far, before the patient continues. As in the case of requests for repair, requests for confirmation orient their recipients to a last item rather than a next item in a series of events.

A third class of conditionally relevant question-types is composed of items Schegloff (1981) called *surprise markers* (such as "Really?" "Oh Really?" "Izzat so?"[7]). Often, these appear in the aftermath of some bit of "news" delivery, in places where simple acknowledgment tokens might fail to convey a sufficiently emphatic display of the listener's appreciation:

(Dyad 1:230–248)

    Patient: .hh Would it be a good idea tuh take prescri:pshuns,
              exdra prescripshuns along, d'yuh think they'd be
              ho:nored in Europe?

                        .
                        .   ((13 lines deleted))
                        .

    Physician: I- they wouldn' even honor my priscipshun in
               Alabama
    Patient: Oh ⌈ri:lly?   ⌉
    Physician: ⌊Much less- ⌋   (.) Hungary.

Just above, the physician continues rather than replying to the patient's (overlapped) surprise marker. While the doctor may not have heard the patient's "ri:lly?" (since both were speaking simultaneously), a lack of response is typical for items such as this one. Surprise markers used with interrogative intonations can only invite confirmation or disconfirmation of the objects preceding them (e.g., "Yes, really!" or "No, I was kidding!"). Thus, even where responses to surprise markers might occur, it is clear that they will be aimed at prior objects in a sequence.

The analysis presented in Chapter 5 excluded conditionally relevant question-types from the general category of "questions" that call for "answers." Since these items appear to look backward rather than forward in sequential time, they seem to be dependent on some equivalent of a first pair part for their intelligibility.[8] However, though conditionally relevant queries may not properly be counted as "questions," an independent analysis of their organization provides the opportunity to address problems of hearing and understanding as topics in their own right. Where the use of questions is constrained by speaker identities (cf. Frankel, in press b), the use of more subtle forms may assume added importance in guaranteeing mutual intelligibility. So, while patient-initiated questions may be dispreferred in medical encounters, conditionally relevant question-types offer alternative and perhaps less obtrusive methods for managing mishearings and misunderstandings between patients and family physicians.

MEDICAL MISFIRES

In the 21 encounters in this collection, I identified all conditionally relevant question-types on the basis of the criteria specified above. Thus, I included all requests for confirmation of a prior utterance (assertions to which "Like . . . ?" "Yuh know?" "Right?" or "Okay?" were appended), requests for repair of a prior utterance (interrogative question terms, complete or partial repetitions or "Y'mean . . . ?" coupled with candidate understandings of prior speech objects), and markers of surprise at prior utterances ("Izzat right?" "Really?" or "Ye:ah?"). Given that many of the lexical items used in conditionally relevant queries are employed for other interactional purposes too,[9] I wanted to include only those requests and markers that exhibited a clear conditional relevance on actual prior speech objects. So, ambiguous instances (e.g., the presence of an "Okay" or "Yuh know" without an interrogative intonation pattern) were omitted from coding and subsequent analysis.

A second analytical task involved classification of responses to these question-types. As we have seen, one criterion for distinguishing them from "questions" per se is the sort of response (if any) they are likely to produce. For example, if surprise markers are employed to show emphatic appreciation rather than posing actual queries, we would expect to find fewer "answers" in their wake than in the wake of "questions" per se. Moreover, if requests for confirmation simply provide opportunities for responses (rather than demanding them), we would expect to find some opportunities not taken and others used to disconfirm that for which ratification was sought. Inasmuch as rejoinders to conditionally relevant question-types (and to questions generally) can consist of simple acknowledgment tokens (e.g., "Uh-huh," "Mm-hmm," or "Yeah"), nonverbal responses (e.g., nods or lateral headshakes) were also considered rejoinders when they appeared to be treated that way by participants.[10]

Table 4 presents the overall distribution of conditionally relevant question-types between physicians and patients in this collection. In the 21 exchanges and 532 pages of transcript, a total of 251 such queries were observed. Of this total, 55 percent (138) were initiated by physicians; 45 percent (113) were initiated by patients. Hence, the distribution of these items between physicians and patients is virtually symmetrical.[11]

Total question-types in each category show a broad range. Requests for confirmation appeared nearly twice as often (144) as requests for repair (76), and markers of surprise occurred least frequently of all three types (31). But, within each category of conditionally relevant query, the distribution of initiations approaches symmetry between doctor and patient. Patients ventured 47 percent of all requests for confirmation (versus physicians' 53 percent), 41 percent of all requests for repair (versus physicians' 59 percent), and 48 percent of all surprise markers (versus physicians' 52 percent). In these exchanges, then, doctors and patients were essentially equally likely to request confirmation, request repair, and produce markers of surprise at prior utterances.

The symmetry of these patterns is highlighted when initiations of conditionally relevant queries are compared with initiations of "questions" per se. As we saw in Chapter 5, these patients posed only 9 percent (68) of the total (773) questions asked. Yet, they initiated nearly half of (113) the conditionally relevant queries. Thus, the dispreference for patient-initiated questions observed earlier does not appear to hold for conditionally relevant queries. While patients may hesitate to ask direct questions of their doctors, they exhibit little (if any) reluctance to use interrogative forms for less obtrusive purposes.[12]

Doctors' and patients' responses to conditionally relevant queries

TABLE 4
Conditionally Relevant Question-Types
in Encounters between Physicians and Patients

Question-Type	Percentage of Physician-Initiated Queries	Percentage of Patient-Initiated Queries	Total
Requests for Confirmation[1] of Prior Utterances	53 (77)	47 (67)	100 (144)
Requests for Repair[2] of Prior Utterances	59 (45)	41 (31)	100 (76)
Markers of Surprise[3] at Prior Utterances	52 (16)	48 (15)	100 (31)
Totals	55 (138)	45 (113)	100 (251)

1. For example, assertions to which "Like. . . ?", "Y'know?", or "Okay?" are appended.
2. For example, "Hunh?", "What?", or "Pardon?"
3. For example, "Really?", "Is that right?", or "Ye::ah?"

offer further evidence of the distinctive status of these speech objects. Recall that Schegloff and Sacks (1974) described the organization of questions and answers as that of adjacency pairs: Answers are "preferred" in the turns following questions. In fact, the absence of an answer in a turn following a question is a *noticeable* absence, furnishing the "grounds for repetition of the [Q]uestion or some inference based on the absence of an answer" (Schegloff, 1972:77). As seen in Chapter 5, empirical evidence for answers' preferredness is exhibited in these exchanges. Although patients answered physicians' questions more often than the reverse, 96 percent of questions (748 of the total 773) elicited answers from their recipients.

For conditionally relevant queries, however, a different pattern emerges. Of the total 251 question-types that were posed, only 64 percent (160) elicited rejoinders. Further, the response patterns of doctors and patients were virtually identical: 63 percent of patients' queries and 65 percent of physicians' queries produced responses.

To be sure, different question-types elicited different response rates. For example, in the preceding section I suggested that surprise markers might understandably fail to evoke rejoinders from their recipients. If these question-types simulate inquiries to convey emphatic or upgraded appreciation of "news," then responses to such queries might be seen as "responses to responses." In light of the data here presented, this perspective is perhaps warranted: 60 percent of patients' surprise markers (9) and 75 percent of physicians' surprise markers (12) failed to receive responses from their recipients.

On the other hand, requests for repair of others' utterances did generally evoke rejoinders in subsequent turns. Patients in this collection, who answered 98 percent of "questions" asked them by doctors, produced repairs of their own prior utterances in response to 87 percent of the total (45) physician requests. Physicians, who responded to 87 percent of patients' "questions," furnished repairs of their own utterances in response to 77 percent of the (31) patient requests. So, while requests for repair appear somewhat less likely than "questions" to elicit rejoinders, it is clear that both questions and repair requests are likely to evoke some form of response. Recall, however, that responses to these requests (e.g., "Hunh?") consist of actual reiterations of one's own prior utterance or minimal tokens to acknowledge another's candidate understanding (guess) of it (e.g., "Y'mean your hip?"—"Um-hmm").

For analytical purposes of this chapter, responses to requests for confirmation may constitute the most interesting category of reply. In contrast to requests for repair (which elicit recipients' repetitions of their own prior utterances), requests for confirmation invite recipients to respond to prior utterances produced by the *initiators* of such requests. In this sense, a request for confirmation can be seen as the mirror image of a surprise marker: The marker of surprise *offers* a listener's response (e.g., "Rea::lly?"), whereas the request for confirmation *asks for* it (e.g., "It hurts, okay?"). Hence, this particular conditionally relevant question-type furnishes its user the greatest freedom to *invite* expressions of mishearing, misgiving, or misunderstanding from recipients. The use of surprise markers is constrained by the fact that these items approximate forms of response to others' utterances; the use of repair requests is restricted by the preference for self-repair over other repair (Schegloff et al., 1977).[13] However, requests for confirmation can solicit acknowledgment of virtually any prior assertions (be they suggestions, criticisms, or complaints).

The distribution of responses to requests for confirmation in these data also exhibited symmetrical patterns between physicians and patients. Sixty-four percent of patient requests elicited replies from physicians (43 out of 67), while 57 percent of physician requests elicited patient replies (44 out of 77). In response to most requests for confirmation (77 percent) both doctors and patients offered minimal acknowledgment tokens (e.g., "Um-hum" or "Yeah"). But patients—more often than doctors—responded to these requests with replies that failed to confirm that for which ratification was sought. In only two (of 67) instances were patients' requests for confirmation met with doctor rejoinders that withheld ratification of patients' prior utterances.[14] In eight (of 77) instances, doctors' requests for confirmation received patient rejoinders which failed to confirm the physicians' prior utterances.

Assuredly, the numbers of replies that failed to confirm are exceedingly small (constituting only 3 percent of physician rejoinders and 10 percent of patient rejoinders to requests for confirmation). And "failure to confirm" is often, as we shall see, a subtle method of withholding ratification rather than an explicit expression of disagreement. But, given our current knowledge of the nature of the physician-patient relationship, we would expect patients to resort to such delicate means of expressing potential misgivings and misunderstandings to their physicians. If, by way of analogy, physicians stand in relation to patients as entities "not to be questioned," then patients' methods of negotiating queries with them should be subtle ones indeed. For just this reason, patients' vehicles for withholding ratification deserve more detailed attention. Thus, the section below offers a qualitative analysis of patients' failures to confirm in response to doctors' invitations.

MISHEARINGS, MISGIVINGS, AND MISUNDERSTANDINGS

As noted earlier, requests for confirmation consist of otherwise declarative utterances to which query terms are appended. Elsewhere (West and Zimmerman, 1977), I suggest that the time slot allocated to a current speaker is potentially two things. First, it is an interval in which a speaker may also engage in some nonverbal activity (e.g., conducting an examination). Second, it is an interval in which a speaker's utterance may itself unfold as a recognizable action (e.g., as a suggestion, bit of advice, or piece of instruction).[15]

The physicians in this collection tended to append query terms to utterances which otherwise might be seen as explanations, advisements or proposals for future action. So, when their requests were successful in evoking confirmation from patients, the process of ex-

plaining, advising, or planning unfolded as a conjoining activity *be-*
tween physician and patient:

(Dyad 4:236–241)

Physician: si:t do:wn (.6) at the ta:ble, an' eat (.) slo::w, an' .h
            make sure yuh taste ev'ry single bite cha put in the
            mou::th- in yer mou:th = don't let a bite go by:: .h that
            cha don' remember, okay? ((sniff! blowing her nose))
                              (.4)
Patient: Yeah.

In this fragment, for example, what might otherwise be seen as a set
of instructions (or "doctor's orders") are transformed by the patient's
confirmation into a jointly ratified plan between physician and
patient.[16]

Inasmuch as physicians command authority in matters of health
and illness in our culture (cf. Parsons, 1951), the conversion of their
instructions into "requests" and "confirmations" might seem strange,
or at best, unnecessary. However, requests for confirmation, in paro-
dying "questions," invite second parts—the confirmations themselves.
And their provision of opportunities for response facilitates the possibility of ongoing mutually intelligible talk between speakers. As
Schegloff and Sacks (1974) observe, "It is through the use of adjacent
positioning that appreciations, failures, correctings, et cetera, can
themselves be understandably attempted" (p. 240). Hence, it is in the
aftermath of these requests that one would look for evidence of mishearings, misgivings, and misunderstandings.

To assess such evidence, we might begin by remembering that most
responses to requests for confirmation (77 percent) consisted of minimal acknowledgment tokens (e.g., "Yeah," "Uh-hmm" or their nonverbal substitutes). Given this, we can appreciate the strangeness of
such nonverbal "rejoinders" as are illustrated in the following
fragments:

(Dyad 4:442–446)

Physician: Ay:::e- checked in:ta that:t, oka::y? and:::d-
            (1.0) No:t no::t- extensively, I didn't search all the
            lidd'chure:, =

Patient:	= ((clears throat))
	(.4)

(Dyad 4:500–508)

Physician: Let's stay on- uh::: what we're doin' right no:w. Okay?
((she sits down again)) No:w. The PILLS yer takin'
right now. Yer takin' this one ((rattling the bottle of
pills))
(.)
Patient: .hh-hh ((it sounds as if he is sitting down next to her
again, and the chair scrapes))
Physician: Izzat right?
Patient: ((clears throat))
Physician: Izzat the one . . .

The fragments are taken from a larger stretch of talk in which this
(Black male) patient questions his white female physician about his
high blood pressure medicine (see Chapter 4). The patient has indicated he is worried about possible carcinogenic effects of the medication; the doctor has indicated that continuation of the medication is
the best alternative presently available. Note that the doctor's initial
request for confirmation ("Ay:::e- checked in:ta tha:t, oka::y?") is followed shortly by a pause, rather than an acknowledgment token from
the patient. Instead, the physician's qualifying comment ("I didn't
search all the lidda'chure:") is immediately appended by the patient's
clearing of his throat.

To be sure, throats do require occasional clearing, especially in
preparation for speaking. However, the patient does not begin speaking after clearing his throat in the first fragment, nor does he do so
in the interval of silence that follows his nonverbal production. Further, in the second fragment, the doctor's next attempt at eliciting
confirmation ("Let's stay on- uh::: what we're doin' right now:.
Okay?") again evokes no response from the patient. And when she
presses the matter ("Yer takin' this one . . . Izzat right?"), the patient
chooses that moment to clear his throat again. Here too, his throat
clearing is not followed by the beginnings of speech.[17]

Since requests for confirmation solicit, rather than demand, recipients' responses, a lack of response does not necessarily disconfirm

that for which ratification is invited. But a response that consists of something *other* than an acknowledgment indeed fails to confirm any activity being proposed by a prior utterance. Hence, the patient's throat clearing in precisely the slot in which confirmation could occur constitutes at least a lack of ratification (by the patient) of the doctor's proposal. Elsewhere in this encounter, discussion of the controversial medication is finally resolved with yet another nonverbal production by the patient (see also Chapter 4).

(Dyad 4:471–479)

Physician: <u>If I</u> brought cha some <u>arduchul</u>(s) saying thet this wuz
        Okay:::, would juh bih<u>lie</u>:::ve me? .h
                            (1.0)
Patient: Ye:ah, su:re, defin ⌈at'ly.
                         ⌊OKa:y.⌋
                          (.)
Physician: O ⌈kay:,   ⌉ o::kay. =
Patient: ⌊But u:h-⌋   = ((clears throat)) .h Whether
         I would cha:nge to it'r no:t it would be a diff-
         y'know, a nuther thi::ng,

Here, the clearing of the patient's throat is latched to a nearly explicit refusal to follow the doctor's advice (he might "believe" the physician if she brought him some articles supporting her opinion, but whether or not he would follow her advice "would be a nuther thi::ng.") In light of this patient's repeated failures to confirm in response to the physician's requests, such as resolution of the matter is perhaps not surprising.

From such subtle displays as misplaced throat clearings, we can turn to more overt verbal responses that constitute failures to confirm. Consider the following excerpts:

(Dyad 8:540–554)

Physician: Mister Fea:thers here is gonna- (.) .h gonna:
        help you so- (.) you can pass yer urine the
        right ⌈wa:y, OKay?   ⌉
Patient: ⌊((cough, cough⌋ drinking a large glass of water))

Physician: Thure's a speshul way we gotta do it fer this
test, = ah'm jus' gonna look ad it under the
micruhscope. .h It's be:en a long time since we've
looked ad it.

(.2)

Patient: Ye:ah, 'ull ((from behind water glass))

(.2)

Physician: Okay?

(.4)

Patient: Wull ah ha- ah sometimes when I ha- ah, see- ah ha-
hadda take a great big drinka wadder that big,
((holding up his hands to show a larger size than the
cup he's using)) .hh an' then- then ah don't have no
trouble with goin' duh the ba:throom, it goes- .hh
soo:n, but you know:, there's only a half hour.

(Dyad 10:1017–1021)

Patient: Here's some moah a that- blastud med'cine.

(.2)

Physician: h. Now just hang o::n the:re, ((helping the patient to
sort through her pills)) you only go:t about six more
months tuh go:::. (.2) Right? =

Patient: = 'Bout 'ei:ght.

(Dyad 6:605–610)

Physician: I: percei::ve fro:m you: tha:t ( ) yer att:itude i:s
thet = we:ll, ((begins affecting a quavering voice, as if
feeble)) these o::ther discs mi:ght be a littul wea:k.
(1.0) yuh ⎡ know::? ⎤
Patient: ⎣ Wull = I'm ⎦ not saying tha:t now,
Docktuh Mea:d said that.

In each of these fragments, the patient's response to the physician's
request for confirmation is composed of something *other* than a minimal acknowledgment token (i.e., "Ye:ah, wull . . . ," "Bout ei:ght,"
and "Wull = I'm not saying tha:t"). Thus, in each excerpt, we can
observe a patient failure (or, in one case, a refusal) to confirm that for
which ratification was sought (i.e., "You can pass yer urine that right

wa:y," "Now just hang o::n the:re," and "Yer att:itude i:s thet these o::ther discs mi:ght be a littul we:ak"). And, as is evident in the first excerpt (from Dyad 8), rejoinders which offer something other than confirmation may have pronounced consequences for subsequent talk. In that excerpt, the patient escalates his "Yes, well" response to a lengthy explanation regarding his inability to produce a urine sample.

More serious, though, are the potential consequences of failures to confirm for the larger scale activities being conducted as these exchanges transpire.[18] While talking with patients, doctors are simultaneously involved in formulating diagnoses, treatment plans, and courses for future action. If patients' failures to confirm are not noticed by their doctors, physicians can miss valuable pieces of information that might assist them in their formulations. Thus, the physician who is under the impression that his patient has only six (rather than eight) months remaining on "that blastud med'cine" might neglect to add such encouragement as the patient needs to complete her course of treatment. The physician who fails to notice his patient's misgivings regarding his ability to produce a urine sample might well end up not getting one (especially consequential in this case, where the patient is a diabetic). And the doctor who remains erroneously convinced that his patient's back problem is a matter of his "attitude" might not continue to provide health care for that patient for much longer.

Consider, in the final example just below, the possible consequences of a patient's failure to confirm:

(Dyad 4:346–364)

Physician: An' tho:se 'r the diffrun' foo:d groups 't yuh wanna try
            duh ge:t. .h Y'know, go light- .hh An' they a:ll- have
            nutrishunal val:ue for you, .h an' you nodice that
            swee:ts aren' on that li:st at a:ll. OKay?
                        (.2)
Patient: ((sniff)) O:h, yuh god fru:it here, right? .h=
Physician: =Um-hmm: (1.0) Insteada havin' a Pepp'
            ⌈ ridge Farm: coo::   ⌉ kie,=
Patient: ⌊ Ah don' eat a lodda fruit. ⌋
Physician: = .h Yuh c'n ha:ve an awr::unge, .h
                        (1.2)

Patient: ⎛ Ah do:n'-   ⎞
Physician: ⎝ y'know, which ⎠ has calories, in it but it has so:me
nutrishunal value too. .hh But the thin:g i::s Mister
Muhlloy, .h I don't wan' cha duh deNY: yerself

.
.
. ((three lines deleted))
Doctor: Whudda yuh sa:y
(.)
Patient: Mm: 't's okay:

In fact, the physician's proposed diet plan is *not* okay. Its major aim is substitution of a food about which the patient is less than enthusiastic ("O:h yuh god fru:it here"). For a patient who does not eat "a lodda fruit," the substitution of an "awr::unge" for a Pepperidge Farm cookie will probably be less than satisfactory. Consequently, the diet plan may be less than successful. As readers of the transcript (rather than participants to the actual encounter), we of course have access to certain disconfirming materials that may have passed unheard by the doctor while she was actually speaking with this patient. For example, both the patient's disparagements of fruit occur in states of simultaneous talk ("Ah don' eat a lodda fruit . . . Ah do:n'-"). But the patient's initial rejoinder to the doctor's request for confirmation is produced in the clear—and it consists of something other than an acknowledgment token. So, even without the patient's subsequent disparagements, it is evident that he has failed to confirm the doctor's proposed course of action.

Throughout the 21 encounters, requests for confirmation were employed to produce jointly ratified explanations, plans, and future courses of action. The two-part coupling of these requests with rejoinders that acknowledged and confirmed activities appeared to facilitate speakers' mutual understanding and validation. More important still, the adjacent positioning of requests and responses offered participants ongoing opportunities for the expression of misgivings, mishearings and misunderstandings. Thus, where patients' responses failed to confirm at physicians' requests, I was able to identify potential miscommunications *as they actually occurred*. In contrast to research methodologies that employ retrospective means of eliciting "trouble" the analysis affords the researcher (and the participants themselves)

an empirically grounded way to recognize mishearings and misunderstandings in the course of their production.

Below, I consider the possible implications of these findings for
issues of greater patient satisfaction, patient compliance and the potential for symmetry in the physician-patient relationship.

GAPS IN DOCTOR-PATIENT COMMUNICATION

The problem of dissatisfaction with the delivery of medical care in the
U.S. is not solely a matter of inadequate financing or insufficient facilities and personnel . . . Of the various factors that tend to contribute to
this discontent, certainly one of the most important is poor communication between doctor and patient. (Korsch and Negrete, 1972:66)

In spite of widespread concern over problems of mutual intelligibility between doctors and patients, few practical solutions to the
problems have been found. As noted earlier in this chapter, much
previous research has relied on retrospective means of eliciting misunderstandings from participants in medical encounters. Through
such methods as post-visit interviews, quizzes, and questionnaires,
physicians' and patients' miscommunications have only been discovered in the wake of the exchanges in which they occurred. Outside
the confines of research designs, however, doctors and patients must
assess one another's responses to words that they use by observing the
other's reactions to them on the spot.

Whereas the use of questions is sometimes advanced as a way to
deal with problems of mutual intelligibility between speakers, in medical dialogues this "solution" appears to pose problems of its own. For
example, my analysis of questions and answers found only 9 percent
of questions were initiated by patients during routine visits to
physicians.

However, physicians also risk a great deal when mutual understanding eludes their patients and themselves. Since mis-diagnoses,
mis-treatments and charges of malpractice are among the possible
outcomes of medical misunderstandings, it seemed reasonable to sup-
pose that some alternative to direct questions must be available to
physicians and patients to ensure their mutual intelligibility. Thus,
this chapter extended the previous analysis of "questions" and "an-

swers" to a further study of the organization of conditionally relevant question-types in medical encounters.

As we have seen, the distributions of these queries differ markedly from the distribution of "questions." While patient-initiated questions appeared to be strongly dispreferred in these exchanges, patients' requests for confirmation, repair, and markers of surprise were not. Fewer conditionally relevant queries than "questions" were observed in these data (251 versus 773, respectively). But patients posed nearly half (45 percent) the total question-types that were initiated. Hence, conditionally relevant queries appear to offer an alternative means of establishing hearing and understanding between doctors and patients which is symmetrically distributed and mutually accessible.

One possible implication of these results pertains to the use of "jargon" in medical dialogues. Although technical terminology is a recurrent complaint in many investigations of patient satisfaction and compliance, research on its effects has yielded inconclusive, and sometimes confusing findings (cf. Ley, 1983). Only two clear threads of consensus emerge from the existing literature: Patients do not like medical jargon and physicians do not know what constitutes it. From the contradictory findings of previous research on this matter (e.g., Korsch and Negrete, 1972; McKinlay, 1975; Wallen et al., 1979 as well as others reviewed in Chapter 2), the physician attempting to improve communication with patients probably will not learn whether to upgrade or downgrade the level of technical terminology employed in actual patient visits. Moreover, as Frankel (forthcoming) notes, whether or not physicians deliberately intend to deceive, obscure, or limit the flow of information to patients, "How the patient actually behaves or receives dominating or limiting communication from the physician, and, of course the physician's subsequent response, is left unaddressed as a topic or focus for research" (p. 26, fn. 8).

The question-types analyzed in this chapter offer an empirically grounded method for assessing the impact of "jargon" on the actual occasions of its use. Thus, where patients' use of surprise markers conveys the receipt of "news," we might look to see what sorts of prior utterances by physicians constituted reports of events or conditions not previously known to their patients. Where patients' requests for repair appear in the wake of physicians' instructions, we might look to see whether simple mishearing of utterances is all that is at issue (cf. Meehan, 1981). And, where physicians' requests for confirmation elicit patient responses that withhold ratification of plans, we might examine patients' response for evidence of understanding of that for which ratification is sought. For example:

(Dyad 10:480–483)

```
Physician:  .h Alri:ght. I think you've jus' got some-
            (.) bursi::dus there. Oka:y?
   Patient: .hh hhh Ah've ha:d- had bursi:dus in muh shoul:der
            buhfo:re. (.4) Bud I never had anything (.6) (much)
            like this,
```

Here, the physician's appended request provides an opportunity for the patient to confirm her understanding of his diagnosis ("you've jus' got some- bursi::dus there"). Simultaneously, the patient is furnished the opportunity to display her understanding of the terminology in which the diagnosis is couched ("Ah've had bursi:dus buhfo:re:). In this way, the analysis of conditionally relevant question-types provide a systematic method for pinpointing mishearings and misunderstandings of technical terms in the course of their actual production.

A further implication of these results pertains to the as yet unexplored possibility of substituting conditionally relevant queries for "questions" in physician-patient talk. Recall, for example, that Frankel's (in press) analysis of over 3,500 utterances produced in medical dialogues found 99 percent of free-standing utterances were initiated by physicians. Of these, the vast majority were doctor-initiated questions. If some conditionally relevant queries (e.g., requests for confirmation) might be used as replacements for doctor-initiated questions, it is at least conceivable that the structure of medical dialogues might assume less interrogative (and more symmetrical) proportions between physicians and patients. Since these question-types tended toward symmetrical distributions in the exchanges analyzed here, it would seem that their use is not constrained by speakers' identities. So, instead of constructing an order of medical exchange in which doctors ask the questions and patients respond to them, physicians and patients might utilize these devices to create a structure of talk affording them further possibilities for a two-way flow of information.

Finally, these results seem to suggest a means of avoiding some medical misunderstandings well in advance of their occurrence. For example, many analysts have remarked on the tendency for patients to avoid mentioning primary reasons for their visits to doctors until relatively late in exchanges with them (Byrne and Long, 1976; Browne and Freeling, 1976; M. A. Stewart et al., 1975).[19] Byrne and Long's analysis of 1,000 medical interviews found a statistically significant number of patients produced some variant of "By the way, doctor" during the last, or next to last, stage of the exchange. Patients' use of "By the way, doctor" and "While I'm here, doctor" tended to be an enormous source of frustration to their physicians, since it often prefaced—all too late—the real, or main, or most emotionally-charged, reason for the visit in the first instance.

In contrast, Byrne and Long observe that doctors' frequent use of "Is there anything else?" and "Do you have any questions?" as devices to invite patients' questions in the terminal stages of visits were not at all successful in producing their stated aims. For 99 out of 100 cases, physicians elicited nothing else at all, and both patient and doctor were up out of their chairs within seconds (p. 57). These particular physician-initiated questions would appear to have become "empty" civilities in most instances—they are not even evocative of patients' "By the ways."

Conditionally relevant queries may offer potential solutions to such difficulties. For example, throughout the initial stages of medical dialogues, physicians are in fact constructing particular sorts of relationships with their patients through what they say and the way in which they say it. If, as findings reported in previous chapters indicate, that relationship consists of an asymmetrical exchange between interviewer and interviewee, it is perhaps not surprising that there is never "anything else" by the time physicians get around to soliciting it. By then, patients may have learned their place.

However, the turn-by-turn organization of sequencing in talk affords an ongoing set of opportunities to convey (and invite) expressions confirming mutual intelligibility between interactants (see Sacks et al., 1974). Both utterances and topics of talk are developed on a turn-by-turn basis, such that the relevance of any "next" utterance is contingent on that of a prior utterance. Hence, Sacks (1972) observes that complaints regarding interruption (e.g., "Wait," "I wasn't finished yet," etc.) must be made in the turns immediately adjacent to their occurrence if they are to be effective. But voicing a complaint also constitutes changing the topic at that point in talk. So, speakers interrupted in the course of their topical development may hesitate to complain about it, since a complaint may itself further delay or obscure topic development.

In the case of medical dialogues, an analogous situation can be noted. Patients whose speech is restricted in answering physician's questions may find few opportunities to pose questions of their own:

> . . . Sequences which routinely restrict speaker-types and turn-types may constitute a system of exchange in which one party (a questioner) recurrently imposes upon another party (an answerer), a set of sequential obligations, the net effect of which is to create a type of deference structure. (Frankel, in press b:6)

But patients whose speech is used to produce jointly ratified explanations, plans, and future courses of action with their physicians may find ample opportunities to deal with "unhearings," misgivings, and misunderstandings *before* they constitute threats to the physician-patient relationship.

SUMMARY AND CONCLUSIONS

Although medical misunderstandings have preoccupied researchers for the past several decades, most investigations have relied on retroactive methods of analysis. Hence, findings have offered doctors and patients few practical guidelines for identifying problems of hearing and understanding as they occur in ongoing talk.

My analysis of conditionally relevant queries between physicians and patients suggests an empirically grounded way of recognizing, and potentially resolving, misunderstandings in medical encounters. Though these findings are of a preliminary nature, based on a non-random sample of patients and family physicians, they indicate that doctors and patients have mutually accessible means for establishing intelligibility of their utterances. Thus, the potential for symmetry in the physician-patient relationship may be much greater than has been previously supposed.

CHAPTER 7

Laughter and Sociable Commentary in Medical Encounters*

Over a decade has passed since Barbara Korsch and her colleagues issued their now-classic descriptions of problems associated with doctor-patient communication (Francis, et al., 1969; Freeman et al., 1971; Korsch and Negrete, 1972). Several of these problems have become topics of considerable research in subsequent years; for example, physicians' use of abstract technical jargon, their failures to elicit primary complaints from patients, and patients' failures to ask questions of their doctors. However, other "gaps" in communication between physicians and patients have received little, if any, attention since they were first identified.

For example, Korsch and Negrete's (1972) study of pediatric interviews in a large teaching hospital (reviewed in earlier chapters) found "less than 6 percent of the doctor's communication to the mother carrie[d] positive affect (in the form of friendly remarks, joking, agreement [or] support)" (pp. 73–74). Instead, physicians' contributions tended to consist of "neutral informational statements" (p. 73), and they were rarely interspersed with such commonplace courtesies as introductions, greetings, or the use of patients' names. Korsch and

*A preliminary report of the laughter analysis, "Doctor-Patient Dialogues: No Laughing Matters," by Candace West and Sofia Gruskin, was presented at the Annual Conference of the International Communication Association, Boston, Mass., 1982. A subsequent report, "Positive Affect, Negative Effect: Laughter and Sociable Commentary between Doctors and Patients," by Candace West, was presented at the Society for the Study of Social Problems Annual Meeting, Detroit, 1983.

Negrete observed that the use of these civilities generally produced positive results, despite a widespread belief in the need for social distance between physician and patient (e.g., Parsons, 1951; 1975; Davis, 1968; or Leventhal, 1965).

In the last ten years, most researchers still have excluded "sociable" exchange from serious consideration in investigations of physician-patient communication.[1] Some analysts explicitly exempt what they term "miscellaneous, or social, comments" from their study designs (e.g., Waitzkin and Stoeckle, 1976; Waitzkin, 1979; Wallen et al., 1979). Others (such as Byrne and Long, 1976) view such items as parts of "patient preliminaries" (nonconsequential niceties that occupy 10–15 seconds prior to the real business at hand). As we saw in Chapter 6, even "normal troubles"—which abound in virtually any form of speech exchange—tend to be excluded from research on medical encounters. In short, the civilities which make for friendly conversation are the phenomena least attended to in investigations of doctor-patient encounters.[2]

The aim of this chapter is to provide an explicit empirical examination of sociable interaction between patients and family physicians during routine visits to the doctor. At issue here are those little mundane civilities that are generally regarded as the "social cement" of friendly discourse: laughter, salutations, and the mutual exchange of names. My analysis of laughter suggests that this aspect of sociable exchange is organized in asymmetrical distributions between parties in medical encounters. Patients, as we shall see, volunteer laughter more readily than doctors, but their "invitations to laugh" (see below) have a much lesser likelihood of acceptance than do those of physicians. With regard to naming practices, further asymmetries emerge: Physicians address patients in familiar terms that patients do not reciprocate. However, closer inspection of the local contexts in which address terms are employed (e.g., greetings and introductions) indicates more intricate dynamics are involved in these patterns than are presupposed in existing descriptions of them. Although patients call their doctors by title and surname more often than the reverse, the most common medical encounter is one in which neither party calls the other by any name at all. I discuss the implications of these findings in a concluding section, addressing the import of sociable conversation for the physician-patient relationship.

LAUGHTER AND ITS COROLLARIES

To analyze laughter as a socially negotiated matter necessitates some means of identifying "who started it." Identification per se would seem an easy task; everyone knows that laughter is something that follows a "joke" and a "joke" is something that gets laughed at. This commonsensical approach is taken in most studies of humor, where those possessed of "humor" (or a sense of it, at any rate) are identified by the laughter that follows the things they say (see Kramarae, 1981:54–55). Conversely, people without a sense of humor are identified by the absence of laughter in the wake of their would-be witticisms.

One obvious problem with this approach is the confounding of a joke's specification with the subsequent response to it. If "jokes" are those things that get laughed at, there can be no such thing as an unfunny joke. However, even psychoanalytic studies of humor (which are devoted to internal sources of humor's appreciation) recognize that the same joking remarks are not seen as equally funny by everyone. As Coser observed some time ago, "Humor relies on the collective perception of those to whom it is addressed and is therefore defined by the social situation in which it occurs" (1960:81). Thus, she contends that laughing with others presupposes at least some common consensus on a definition of the situation.

Although Coser's refinements lead us away from defining a joke simply as "that which gets laughed at," they offer no systematic means of distinguishing "laughing with" from "laughing at" a would-be joke's teller. For example, most people can recall occasions on which they were made the butts of "jokes" they had not intended to be funny. In these situations, one often has little recourse but to join in "laughing with" others in order to avoid being "laughed at" by them.

Moreover, appreciation of some jokes is apparently limited to particular groups. As Kramarae notes, humor is largely defined within particular cultural contexts, and "much joking is based on ingroup/ outgroup relationships" (1981:52; see also Coser, 1959:172). Hence, "In a reflective analysis of her own childhood, Beatts (1975) writes that by definition all boys in her high school had a sense of humor while girls were thought to have a sense of humor if they laughed when they were the object of the joke" (Kramarae, 1981:57). Such considerations underscore the *analytical* necessity for distinguishing initiations of laughter from subsequent responses to them.

Invitations to Laugh

Recent work by Jefferson (1979) provides an elegant theoretical basis for making just such distinctions. She begins with a deceptively simple observation: "laughing with" is characterized by the presence of two or more parties laughing simultaneously. Thus, instances of single parties laughing alone, after one or another of their utterances, do not constitute instances of "laughing with" co-participants in interaction.

Second, Jefferson notes that actual instances of simultaneous laughter are routinely preceded by one party laughing alone:

> Dan: I thought that wz pretty outta sight didju hear me say'r you a junkie.
>
> (0.5)
>
> Dan: hheh heh
> Dolly: hhheh-heh-heh
>
> (Jefferson, 1979:80)

Here, for example, a *candidate laughable* (" 'r you a junkie") evokes silence (0.5) rather than a response from its recipient. But when its initiator begins laughing himself, the recipient joins in almost instantly.

To be sure, pauses need not intervene between instances of single party laughter and subsequent productions of "laughing with":

> Ellen: He s'd well he said I am cheap he said, .hh about the big things. he says but not the liddle things, hhhHA HA HA HA HA
> Bill: heh heh heh
>
> (Jefferson, 1979:81)

In the fragment just above, Ellen's initiation of laughter is tagged immediately to her completion of an utterance and Bill joins in with no post-completion pause.

Jefferson (1979) observes that any particular utterance may be followed by a variety of responses, and not all utterances call for laughter in their aftermath. Thus, she suggests that on completing utterances that warrant laughter by co-participants, speakers may *in-*

vite laughter by beginning to laugh themselves. Below is a further example of such a laughter invitation and its subsequent *acceptance:*

(Dyad 3:384–389)

```
    Patient:    .hh So we were talkin' about ro:les. (1.2)
                u:hm henh-eh! Gir::ls 'er .hh They we::re
                more chauvinis:tic than the men were!
──────────→ hengh! =
    Physician:        = heh ⎡heh-heh!⎤
    Patient:               ⎣Fe::   ⎦  male chauvini ⎡stic!        ⎤
    Physician:                                      ⎣.engh-.engh⎦
```

Note that just after completion of a candidate laughable ("They we::re more chauvinis:tic than the men were!"), this patient appends his own laughter particle ("hengh!"), and the doctor joins him in laughter within a "syllable" of the laughter invitation. The detailed transcription of laughter particles affords us a microscopic view of this sequentially organized production of "simultaneous" laughter by two parties to talk.

A contrast is provided by examining *declinations* of laughter invitations. Jefferson avers that one cannot reject an invitation to laugh simply by failing to join in. Rather, a declination is achieved by talking over the ongoing production of laughter by another party. Just below, for example, the patient's candidate laughable is followed by a brief pause before her invitation is issued:

(Dyad 10:675–686)

```
    Patient:   Yestidy ah uz- (.) tellin' (.2) Mary, ah giss it wu:z,
                                    (.)
    Physician: Um-hm.
                                    (.)
    Patient:   .h Docktuh Wilbur nevuh ha:s hurt me:.
──────────→ (.4) hunh-hunh-hunh ⎡hunh-hunh! Ye-hunh-hunh⎤ =
    Physician:                    ⎣Now yuh cun tell 'er       ⎦
    Patient:         = ⎡-hunh-hunh. .h!⎤
    Physician:       = ⎣that's not true:!⎦
                          (.2)
```

Patient: .hh! =
Physician: = Climb dow:n, an' put back yer- (.2)
              blou:se on

However, rather than joining her in laughter, the physician talks over
the laughter this patient produces ("Now yuh cun tell 'er that's not
true:!"). Thus, the physician not only fails to "laugh with" the patient,
but also intrudes on her single-party production of laughter with a
candidate substitution of his own (i.e., speech). Speech, notes Jefferson, terminates the relevance of laughter at the point at which it
begins.

To demonstrate the interactional work involved in the social production of laughter, Jefferson invites us to compare instances such as
those above with instances of *voluntary* (i.e., unsolicited) laughter:

(Dyad 14:818–827)

Patient: I lo:ve tuh walk aroun' duh sto:ahs

                              .
                        . ((three lines deleted))
              'n that ki:lls 'im. (1.0) So whud I do:
              with him no::w, .h if I think I may even
              wa:lk aroun' a stoah, is . . . take an'
              si:d 'im in the middle a the maw::ll,
              where 'e cun watch the- (.4) ((patient
              swings her wrist back and forth)) .h
              pri ⎧tty gir:ls walk-   ⎫
Physician: ⎩hengh-hengh-hengh-hengh-⎭ hengh! =
Patient: = Pritty gir:ls walk by.

Here, in response to the telling of a possible joke, the physician volunteers laughter on his own ("hengh-hengh-hengh-hengh"). The patient's repetition of her conclusion in the clear ("Pritty gir:ls walk by")
offers some evidence for the possible equivocal status of her utterance
as a "joke."[3] As analysts of these excerpts, we of course have no way
of determining whether the patient intended her remarks to be
funny; the point is, neither does the physician who is her co-partici-
pant in the interaction. In volunteering laughter as the appropriate
response to her comments (in contrast to other possible responses),

the physician relies on his own determination, minus any invitation from the patient.

To summarize then, laughter produced on a voluntary basis is proffered, rather than invited by its recipient. In contrast, laughter invitations solicit responses, in the form of acceptances (joining in) or declinations (talking over the laughter of the other). Jefferson's analysis provides a theoretically grounded way of identifying instances of laughter that are socially produced between parties to talk. Such seemingly spontaneous occurrences as two people laughing with one another (or one person "happening" to be laughing alone) are thus made available for systematic empirical inspection. So we now have a basis for exploring the results of my own analysis of laughter produced between physicians and patients in this collection.

LAUGHING MATTERS IN MEDICAL DISCOURSE

The 21 encounters were carefully examined to locate instances of laughter by one or both parties to talk, and those instances were then classified according to the criteria specified above. To reiterate, *volunteered* laughter included all those instances which followed another party's verbal or nonverbal production without a production of laughter by that other. And, *invitations to laugh* were distinguished by their post-completion addendums of laughter particles to candidate laughables produced by the initiators of the invitations.[4] Following Jefferson, I categorized *acceptances* as simultaneous productions of laughter following laughter invitations; *declinations* were identified by post-invitational speech over the laughter of initiators. These operational definitions permitted me to distinguish parties "laughing with" others from those "laughing at" them, and to separate instances of parties laughing together from those in which individuals laughed alone.

First, I examined the distribution of laughter produced on a volunteer basis by patients and family physicians in this collection (see Table 5). Patients, in the aggregate, produced 61 percent of the total volunteered laughter I observed, in comparison to physicians' 39 percent. In two-thirds of these encounters (14 of the 21), patients volunteered as much or more laughter than their doctors. To be sure, in the 532 pages of transcript, patients only volunteered laughter on 49 occasions, and physicians on 31. The relative scarcity of voluntary

TABLE 5
Voluntary Laughter in Encounters between
Physicians and Patients

	Percentage of *Physician Laughter*		*Percentage of* *Patient Laughter*	
Black female patient, 16 years	—	(0)	—	(0)
Black female patient, 20 years	—	(0)	—	(0)
White female patient, 36 years	—	(0)	100	(5)
White female patient, 17 years	—	(0)	100	(3)
White female patient, 32 years	—	(0)	100	(2)
White male patient, 36 years	—	(0)	100	(2)
Black male patient, 36 years	—	(0)	100	(1)
White male patient, 16 years	—	(0)	100	(1)
Black female patient, 52 years	14	(1)	86	(6)
Black female patient, 31 years	20	(1)	80	(4)
Black female patient, 67 years	31	(4)	69	(9)
White male patient, 38 years	33	(2)	67	(4)
White female patient, 82 years	33	(2)	67	(4)
White male patient, 56 years	50	(1)	50	(1)
Black male patient, 17 years	60	(3)	40	(2)
White female patient, 53 years	67	(6)	33	(3)
White male patient, 31 years	75	(3)	25	(1)
Black male patient, 58 years	86	(6)	14	(1)
Black male patient, 26 years	100	(1)	—	(0)
White female patient, 58 years	100	(1)	—	(0)
Total	39	(31)	61	(49)

laughter in these dialogues suggests that, in and of itself, doctor-patient talk contains few "laughing matters."

Of course, the distribution of volunteered laughter merely provides us with a rough indication of the incidence of candidate laughables in the eyes of the beholders. It includes instances of laughter following objects which speakers may have intended to be funny, following those which speakers may not have intended to be funny, and following those which may have been only "spuriously" funny from the point of view of the laugher.[5] At present, there is no way to separate these possibilities from one another.

However, Table 6 offers a more detailed picture of the social production of laughter, through a comparison of acceptances and declinations of laughter invitations. As Table 6 illustrates, laughter invitations were refused more often than they were accepted by recipients in these exchanges: 78 percent of physicians' invitations and 94 percent of patients' invitations were declined by their recipients. The "success rate" for doctors' invitations, though, is better than that of patients': Physicians' invitations were accepted in two of the nine instances in which they were initiated, whereas patients' invitations to laugh "succeeded" on only four of the 66 total occasions they were issued.

TABLE 6
Invitations to Laugh in Encounters between
Physicians and Patients

	Percentage of Physician Laughter Invitations	*Percentage of Patient Laughter Invitations*
Invitation Accepted	22 (2)	6 (4)
Invitation Declined	78 (7)	94 (62)
Total	100 (9)	100 (66)

What we see, then, is an unequal distribution of laughter between the physicians and patients in this collection. Physicians invited laughter much less readily than patients, but their laughter invitations had a better likelihood of eliciting acceptances from their recipients. Within these patterns, we can see a distortion of one of the most important social functions of laughter between human beings: "To laugh, or to occasion laughter through humor and wit, is to invite those present to come close. Laughter and humor are indeed like an invitation, be it an invitation for dinner, or an invitation to start a conversation: *it aims at decreasing social distance*" (Coser, 1959:172; emphasis added). Where invitations to "come close" are rarely issued and frequently declined (especially by status superordinates), it is only reasonable to expect perpetuation of social distance between parties to talk.

SOCIABLE COMMENTARY IN MEDICAL DIALOGUES

Obviously, the experience of laughing together constitutes only one aspect of sociable exchange. Among others specified in Korsch and Negrete's (1972) research are greetings, introductions, and the use of people's names. For these exchanges between patients and family physicians, a systematic quantitative analysis of some of these civilities poses technical problems which are produced, in part, by my mode of data collection. Recall that the medical faculty at the Center were the ones who recorded these exchanges (see Chapter 3). All the material contained on the tapes was transcribed, but not all the tapes included the full duration of the exchanges. Sometimes, the recording cut off the first few moments of greetings; other times, the farewells were cut short at the point at which the tapes ended. Given that such things as greetings and farewells occur only once in any given encounter, a few seconds "lost" to technical difficulty can lose the very phenomena under investigation in that exchange.

Moreover, introductions, by definition, occur only once between two people. After their initial meeting with one another, parties are acquainted (however superficially) and presumably have no further use for such courtesies. Thus, a very large number of first visits would have to be sampled in order to derive a representative picture of introductions between physicians and patients in general.

Such considerations preclude a rigorous statistical analysis of greetings, introductions, and terms of address in the exchanges comprising my collection. Despite this limitation, a detailed preliminary examination of these commonplace courtesies suggests some potentially fruitful directions for further research.

Beginning With Names[6]

> The names, labels and phrases employed to "identify" a people may in the end determine their survival. The word "define" comes from the Latin *definire*, meaning to limit. Through definition we restrict, we set boundaries, we name. (Bosmajian, 1974:5)

In our culture (and many others), a single form of address can reflect power or proximity (Brown and Gilman, 1960; Brown and Ford, 1961; Brown, 1965). As Henley (1977) notes, proximity can be displayed through reciprocal use of "familiar" address terms, such as first names, nicknames, or terms of endearment. But power differences can also be expressed through nonreciprocal use between speakers, with the higher-status person employing familiarities that the lower-status individual may not reciprocate: "Thus, the employer is Mr. Gordon, and the employees, Frank and Mary; the teacher is

Professor Black, and the students, Joan and Bob" (Henley, 1977:68; see also Kramer, 1975). The general principle guiding such matters is one of symmetry between equals and asymmetry between persons who are not equals (Goffman, 1967:64).

As noted earlier, the physician-patient relationship is thought to constitute an archetype of asymmetry in our culture, and sociolinguists are fond of using it as an exemplar for discussions of naming practices. Physicians, of course, are characterized as the high-status persons in this relationship, warranting the use of their title plus surname from patients. In this view, patients can expect to be called by their first names—though they cannot reciprocate the familiarity. In spite of the popular appeal of this prototype (see Note 2, this chapter), empirical research on the actual use of address terms between doctors and patients is exceedingly scarce. In fact, of the numerous studies reviewed in earlier chapters, only those of Korsch and her colleagues have included naming practices as objects of explicit analysis.

Between physicians and patients in this collection, naming practices displayed suggestive but complex configurations (see Table 7). For example, in 12 of the 21 recorded exchanges (over half the total), neither doctor nor patient used any term of address in speaking with the other. In two of the 21, patients addressed physicians formally ("Sir" or title plus surname), while physicians used no terms of address. Conversely, in two exchanges, doctors addressed patients by title and surname, while patients used no terms of address. A total of five exchanges evidenced physicians' use of first names in addressing their patients. Of these, four exhibited the prototypical pattern of asymmetry, in which doctors called patients by their first names while patients reciprocated with formal terms of address. In the 532 pages of transcript I analyzed, no patient ever used a physician's first name as a term of address.

The five patients who were called by their first names include one Black female patient (at 16 years of age, one of the youngest in the sample); two Black male patients (36 and 17 years of age, respectively); one white female patient (at 82 years of age, the oldest patient in this collection); and one white male (56 years old and mentally retarded). All of the doctors who used patients' first names as terms of address were white male physicians.

The two patients who were addressed by title and surname include one white male (36 years of age) and one Black male (58 years of age). The white male patient was formally addressed by a white male physician; the Black male patient received this courtesy from a white female physician. It is worth noting that none of the four women physicians was ever addressed formally (title plus surname) by patients in this collection (cf. results of the analysis of turn-taking in these exchanges reported in Chapter 4). Moreover, none of the women physicians ever addressed a patient by first name alone.

In summary, then, we find that coparticipants in these medical encounters generally avoid addressing one another directly. In 17 of the 21 (or 80 percent of the total number), either physician or patient used no name at all for the duration of the interaction. For patients

TABLE 7

Terms of Address in Encounters between
Physicians and Patients

	Term Used By Patient to Physician	Term Used By Physician to Patient
White female patient, 53	No Name	No Name
Black female patient, 31	No Name	No Name
White male patient, 38[1]	No Name	No Name
White female patient, 36	No Name	No Name
Black female patient, 52[1]	No Name	No Name
Black female patient, 20	No Name	No Name
White male patient, 16	No Name	No Name
Black female patient, 67[1]	No Name	No Name
White female patient, 17	No Name	No Name
Black male patient, 26	No Name	No Name
White male patient, 31	No Name	No Name
White female patient, 58	No Name	No Name
White male patient, 16	"Sir"	No Name
White female patient, 32	Title & Surname	No Name
White male patient, 56[2]	Title & Surname	First Name
White female patient, 82	Title & Surname	First Name
Black male patient, 36	"Sir"	First Name
Black male patient, 17	"Sir"	First Name
Black female patient, 16	No Name	First Name
Black male patient, 58[1]	No Name	Title & Surname
White male patient, 36	No Name	Title & Surname

1. This patient visited a female physician; others visited males.
2. This patient is mentally retarded.

in six exchanges, formal address terms were the only ones used to address physicians. However, physicians used patients' first names more than twice as frequently as they used their titles and surnames (in five cases versus two).

The familiarity with which physicians used patients' first names does not appear to be a function of patients' ages. As is evident in Table 7, those patients who were first-named by doctors included the youngest and oldest patients in this collection. Further, although the number of patients addressed by first name is very small, more Black patients than white were so designated by physicians. The only white patients who were addressed familiarly by their doctors were very old and female, on the one hand, and mentally retarded, on the other.[7] Finally, it seems that patients' use of physicians' titles and surnames does not guarantee that their doctors will address them with reciprocal respect. Indeed, of the patients who used such formal terms, none received title and surname in return.

Beyond these general patterns of distribution, the most interesting uses of address terms appeared in the vicinity of particular interactional activities (e.g., salutations, introductions, or deliveries of "news"). Below, I provide a detailed examination of these practices, following an initial consideration of the social significance of "common courtesies."

Local Contexts of Address Terms

To employ a specific term of address, people usually require some minimal information about the object of its use. Although generalized forms abound for opening up talk with previously unacquainted persons ("Hey, *you!*", "Excuse me!", etc.) the utility of particular terms (e.g., "Sir" versus "Ma'am") depends on preliminary inspection at the very least. In addition to displaying ourselves in such ways as can be inspected for evidence of our life stage, life circumstances, ethnicity, and gender, we also offer information which gives others clues as to how to name us. In everyday life, introductions serve as the conventionalized means of exchanging this information.

Where third parties are involved, introductions between two people can, of course, reflect those others' concerns as well. Thus, "Doe," known to both "Smith" and "Jones," may introduce the two to one another. In this instance, the form of address used in presentation may be Doe's choice rather than Smith's or Jones's. But where self-introductions are employed (e.g., in dyadic encounters), a meeting between persons may offer further information as to what each of them *prefers* to be called. So, in the hypothesized meeting of Smith and Jones, the latter may opt between "John" and "Johnny" when introducing himself, minus any intervention by Doe. One caveat must be entered here: In general, the greatest freedom of self-designation is accorded the first party to initiate it. For example, if Smith and Jones are meeting for the first time and Smith appends "Mister" to his surname, then Jones's reciprocal obligations are limited in interactionally meaningful fashion. If he responds with "Mister Jones," he maintains social distance from Smith but implies a basis for equality between them. If he introduces himself as "John," his self-designation may serve to lessen social distance, but it may also serve to display him as the lower-status person in the relationship.

The case of an introduction between a doctor and patient presents one further complication. Patients, by and large, are the initiators of first meetings with doctors. For routine office visits, patients must schedule advance appointments at particular times to occasion introductions to physicians. Moreover, in order to obtain such introductions, patients must volunteer a host of sundry details about themselves and their states of health to whoever schedules their appointments. By the time a physician confronts a particular patient for the first time, a file for purposes of introducing that patient will have already been assembled. In a sense, then, physicians are introduced to patients through a third agent—the medical record—before ever coming face to face with them.[8]

This fact may help to account for the absence of any two-way introductions in the exchanges comprising my collection.[9] Where introductions occurred (in only three of the 21 dyads), they consisted exclusively of physicians' self-presentations to patients:

(Dyad 15:420–437)

Physician: Hello:. hh
                                    (.4)
  Patient: (°Hullo)
Physician: How're you: = ah'm Dock:tur Marr:ah (.4) °An: uh:
            (.4) .h Docktuh Ee:son as:t me du: (.4)
            Come un' speak with yuh a mi:nnut. hh

In this consultation, for example, the physician's self-introduction is latched to his salutation to the patient, allowing no slot for the patient to reciprocate.

Below, the initial salutation itself belies the patient's need for self-introduction:

(Dyad 17:060–061)

Physician: Hi::, Wyl:buh. (.4) ((while looking at the patient's
             feet)) I'm Dock:tuh Keye:lee.

Obviously, where a stranger's salutation includes one's name, there is little need to present oneself officially.

In the third case, the patient's lack of self-designation is again apparent:

(Dyad 18:014–022)

Physician: Hullo dere:!
                         (.2)
  Patient: How yuh do:in'
                         (.2)
Physician: I'm Docktuh Woo:dhouse, how're you. ((standing in
             front of the desk now, setting a folder down on its
             surface. He sits down, opens the folder and is looking
             down at the desk while reading it.))
                         (1.2)
  Patient: °Uh: o::kay.

To be sure, the physician's seeming preoccupation with the patient's medical record in this excerpt makes it unclear who he is greeting (the patient's file or the patient himself). The point, though, is that patients' self-introductions were absent in each of the excerpts here presented. And in each, physicians' introductions of themselves employ their titles plus surnames (surnames are in fact stressed—as indicated by the colons—in all three instances).[10] Finally, each of these fragments shows the physician *initiating* such salutations as transpire in them.

The generality of this pattern in medical discourse by and large is, of course, an empirical question. Only three cases were observed in the 21 total exchanges (the tape of a fourth initial visit began a few seconds after interaction started). But in each of these cases, physicians' self-introductions exhibit a decided preference for title plus surname as their form of address.

Indirect evidence for this preference is also suggested by *references to* physicians in the course of these interactions. For example, from time to time in these encounters, particular subjects of discussion necessitated allusions to doctors not present. Prior medications, operations, and treatment regimens usually required reference to some other physician than the one providing current treatment. When patients initiated such references, they occasionally referred to physicians by surname alone (in four instances), but far more frequently they coupled surnames with physicians' titles (in 28 of the 32 total references). When physicians initiated such references, they consistently alluded to other doctors using title plus surname (in 20 of the 20 total references). Neither physicians nor patients ever referred to a doctor by first name. Hence, even where participants to these medical encounters avoid addressing *one another,* their talk displayed a preference for formal terms in indirect physician references.

The preference for formal terms of address for physicians may help explain the lack of patient introductions in these data. As noted earlier, physicians initiated self-introductions and salutations on entering examining rooms where patients waited for them. The temporal organization of these matters thus affords physicians the greatest freedom of self-designation: As first parties to introduce themselves, they may choose terms of address with less constraint than second parties. Like Jones' situation above, patients' opportunities for self-introductions are limited when they are second parties to initiate them. If patients were to respond to physicians' self-introductions using their own titles and surnames, they might be seen as maintaining social distance or as implying some basis for equality with their doctors.

Where one party in a relationship is the culturally designated dominant party, an attempt at reciprocity by the other might be regarded as evidence of disrespect (e.g., the case of parents and children). Rather than employing first name self-introductions (and *displaying* themselves as the lower-status persons in their relationships with doctors), patients may simply use no names at all. Of course, terms of address were generally avoided by participants in these exchanges.

Thus, an interesting next question posed by these patterns of introduction is: When do physicians and patients employ any names at all
when addressing one another?

Patients' Use of Address Terms

Recall that patients used only formal terms to address the doctors
in this collection. In three instances "Sir" was employed; in another
three, title plus surname was used. For all three cases in which patients used "Sir," the term was employed in answering a physician-
initiated question:

(Dyad 15:445–450)

```
Physician:  NO::W, Ah understa:n' that chew:'ve had
            problum' with yer knee::s fer se::v'rul
            yea:::hs. = hh Izzat cuhre:ck? hh
                        (.2)
Patient:   ⌈°Ye:s sir.⌉
Physician: ⌊.h-.h-.h ⌋ AN::D °eh- (.4) is it cher
            KNEE::S that brought cha i:n he:ah dudha::y?
```

Just above, for example, the physician employs an emphatic pattern
of enunciation with split-second timing (reminiscent of television portrayals of cross-examination) in eliciting a respectful response from
the patient.

Below, a physician-initiated question also prompts the patient's use
of Sir ("°suh"):

(Dyad 17:144–155)

```
Physician:  Du:zzit uh .h hurt cha in one: pertickular
            spot, cha wan' =
Patient:                    = .h Yeah, (.6) right over unnder
            here:: ((touching his left knee cap))
                        (.2)
Physician:  Right on the fron:' p⌈art.          ⌉
Patient:                          ⌊Yes: (°s⌋uh.)
```

It is worth noting that in this excerpt and the one preceding it, physicians addressed as "Sir" previously introduced themselves using

their titles and surnames. Hence, these patients using formal address forms for doctors may be following physicians' tacit directions.

In the third case, "Sir" is again implicated in a (multi-component) physician-initiated query:

(Dyad 6:101–111)

Physician: Um-hm. (2.0) ((sitting back in his chair with his
            hands clasped at his belt line)) Are yuh still
            doin' it?
                              (.2)
Patient: Huh?=.h yeah. Ah'm still takin' u:h (.) uh- t-
            treatmun', yeah. Ah'm still doin' (.) th'
            ex:ercise an' stuff, but u:h (.) ah have:n' been goin'
            down there.
Physician: Where 'r you doing it. At home?=
Patient: =Ye:as, suh.
                              (.6)
Physician: Duh yuh do it ev:ry day?

As seen in Chapter 5, physician-initiated questions were rife in these encounters. Chained questions and multiple-component queries were frequently used in such ways as to turn physician-patient talk into an exchange between an interviewer, on the one hand, and interviewee, on the other. In the case of the latter, "Sir" is perhaps the most appropriate response to the initiator of an interrogation.

Patients' use of doctors' titles and surnames were also found in the vicinity of "special" speech events. For example, one instance of such use actually consisted of an indirect reference by a white female patient:

(Dyad 10:675–679)

Patient: Yestidy ah uz- (.) tellin'- (.2) Mary, ah giss it wu:z,

                    .   ((three lines deleted))
                    .

        .h Docktuh Wilbur nevuh ha:s hurt me:.

Here, "Doctor Wilbur's" title and surname are employed to tell him about a conversation had by the patient with someone else. Since the doctor was the subject of that conversation, the patient must employ *some* term of address to reference him in her telling of it now.

In a second case, the use of a physician's title and surname prefaced a white female patient's delivery of a punchline to an exceedingly unhappy story. The address term is initiated in the course of the patient's account of having been molested by a friend of the family when she was a child:

(Dyad 7:519–525)

> Patient: This guy wuz prob:ably- .hh dy:e wuz eight. .hh! An
> this guy wuz probably twenny one: 'r twenny-two at the
> ti:me. h (1.4) .hh The nex' morning my
> mother = as's = me = whut happun = I = tol:d = 'er- (.2)
> .h as = best = I = could = what = happen' = .hh! .hh-.hh
> So she: w- had my stepdad tell him never duh come
> ba:ck. hh .hh ((clenching both fists, punctuating the
> following utterance)) Docktur Hu:mmel, within three
> weeks after tha:t my stepdad starded in on me::. .hh
> (2.0)
> ((the physician is looking at her now, but issues no
> response))

Here, the patient's delivery of news (that her stepfather "starded in" on her following the incident with the patient and the stepfather's best friend) is marked by an attention-getter (i.e., a summons employing the doctor's title and surname). It is worth noting that the summons and news delivery elicit no response from the physician despite their special marking and the extraordinary nature of the news itself.[11]

Finally, the 56-year-old white male patient who was mentally retarded apparently used his physician's title and surname whenever the doctor called him by name—for example, where the physician delivered "news:

(Dyad 8:012–019)

> Physician: YER BLOO:D SUGAR'S LOOKIN' GREA:T! (1.2)
> REAL:LY GOOD! Geor:ge.

Patient: ZIT LOOKIN'GOOD NO::W? ((getting louder to
          match the doctor's amplitude))
                            (.2)
Physician: Yu:p! (.2) Ab::suhlutely, yer lo- yer doin' we:ll.
                            (.2)
Patient: Do:in' go:od, That's goo:d Dockter Jameson, wull ah'm
          glad a that.

And following the physician's re-entry to the examining room after a
lengthy absence:

(Dyad 8:263–265)

Physician: He:y, George. ((walking over to the examining table))
                            (.)
Patient: He:y, Docktuh Jameuhson.

The only self-initiated use of the doctor's title and surname by this
patient occurred when he was trying to attract the physician's
attention:

(Dyad 8:376–385)

Patient: Wull, yuh see when ma- muh- it goes like this
          sometimes. ((holding his hands over his chest and
          flipping his fingers up and down while craning his
          neck to see the physician))
                            (.4)
Physician: Mm-hmm. ((glances quickly at the patient's face and
          returns to examination of his toes))
                            (.2)
Patient: It goes like this sometimes or like this ((clenches his
          fingers together, but the physician isn't looking)) (.8)
          See: Docktur Jame'son?

Even in the case of this patient (whose mental retardation might lead
some to question his conversational competence), the use of a direct
term of address for a physician seems occasioned by "special"
circumstances.

In short, patients' uses of address terms for physicians displayed

systematic patterns. Formal terms were used, but they were not scat-
tered willy-nilly through patients' speech. Rather, they appeared to be
employed only in the contexts of particular interactional activities:
responding to questions, reporting on other talk, summoning attention and, in the case of the mentally retarded patient, responding to
physicians' use of one's own name.

Physicians' Use of Address Terms
    As noted earlier, physicians also tended to avoid address terms in
these exchanges. But when they did call patients by name, the local
contexts of their use were sometimes similar to those of patients. For
example, physicians employed patients' names as attention-getters:

(Dyad 10:924–928)

Physician: .h No:w, let's do thi:s. .h E:llie, if
              ye:r uh (.) ar:m gits be:dder (.4) with
              ((looking up from the chart he is writing
              on)) the combinations of the injeckshuns an'
              the Mowtrun, (.) .h then ah think (.4) ah
              would suggest that you come see Docktor
              Mo:ss (.) in about a month 'r six wee:ks.

(Dyad 4:176–180)

Physician: It takes a con:scious effort though.
                              (.)
  Patient: At's ri ⌈ght⌉
Physician: ⌊.h ⌋ Mister Muhlloy. It's no:d
              un easy thing = it's easy duh gain weight, isn't it.

In one of the above excerpts, a physician employs a first name (to a
white female), in the other, a title plus surname is used (to a white
male); in both, doctors call patients' attention to what they are in the
process of saying by addressing them by name (cf. Schegloff's [1968]
analysis of summons-answer sequences). Thus, one context in which
physicians employed address terms is similar to that in which patients
used them.
    However, far more frequently, physicians used patients' names in
the course of greeting them or bidding them farewell. For doctors in

this collection, these activities were more likely than any others to involve names for patients:

(Dyad 10:530–531)

Physician: ((entering the examining room again after a few
            minutes' absence)) Oka:y, Miss Ellie.
            Lemme get cha a couple a ban:daids.

In this excerpt, for example, the physician's usual first naming of the 82-year-old white female patient is upgraded slightly by his addendum of "Miss" (the patient was in fact a married woman).[12] His farewell to her, though, reverts to first name alone:

(Dyad 10:1158)

Physician: O:key doe:key! ((holding open the door as the patient
            exits))
                              (3.0)
Physician: Take ca:re, Ellie.

"George," the 56-year-old mentally retarded white male patient, also received his first name as a term of address in the context of such rituals:

(Dyad 8:225–230)

Physician: ((sound of door opening)) AH'LL SEE YUH IN
            MI::NNUT.
                              (.2)
  Patient: .h O::KAY hh
                              (.2)
Physician: OKAY: GEORGE. ((door closes))

A pattern of salutations displayed by one physician in the course of his morning rounds is so striking (and so illuminative of basic sociological concerns) that it warrants more detailed inspection here. This physician was the only one in the collection to be recorded in three separate exchanges with patients. On the morning that these recordings took place, the doctor was off to a late start and was 45 minutes late for his first patient of the day. After meeting briefly with this patient, the physician left the room "momentarily" while the patient disrobed for an examination. Considerably later, he returned to the examining room and greeted the patient in the following fashion:

(Dyad 9:284–287)

Physician: Sor:ry duh keep you waiting Mister Crow:un,

(.4)

Patient: [(°tch S'all raht.)]
Physician: [Hadda li'l prob] lum

Here, the physician's tardy return to the patient is followed by an apology, an explanation for his lateness, and the use of the patient's title plus surname (one of only two such uses observed in the collection as a whole).

Owing, perhaps to the physician's late start and a longer-than-scheduled visit with his first patient, he was 55 minutes late for his second appointment of the morning. On entering the examining room to meet his second patient, the physician opened up the interaction in rather different fashion:

(Dyad 7:005–016)

Physician: Ah'm la:te as u:sual.

(.)

Patient: hh It's alri::ght .hh (.) I broughd a boo:k.
Physician: hh Ye:ah-hhhh ((turning his swivel chair around
            to be seated)) 'D a relatively ma:jor problem
            earlier tuhday hh hh, but.

(.)

Patient: Aw:::a! hh-hh

(.)

Physician: Now:: muh mi:nd i:s- ((he finishes putting papers on
            his desk into a pile)) (.) completely ready fer you:.

In this excerpt, we find an announcement rather than an apology ("Ah'm la:te as u:sual"), and the patient addressed by no name at all. The physician offers an explanation for his tardiness in this case, but here, it "waits" for the patient's acceptance of his apology ("It's alri::ght"). Note that the "l'il problum" alluded to in the first excerpt has become a "relatively ma:jor problem" in this encounter.

The exchange with the second patient took less time than was allocated for it, so by the time this physician met his third patient that morning, he was merely 45 minutes late. In the third encounter, still another opening was used:

(Dyad 6:004–009)

Physician: We:::ll, Le::ster!
                                (.4)
    Patient: °Hmm? ((sitting with one hand on his knee and the
                   other propping up his head, with his arm on the
                   chair rest))
                                (2.6)
Physician: Sor:ry duh keep yuh wai:ting

In this fragment, the patient receives an apology, in the same words as were used with the first patient. But in this exchange, no explanation is proffered, and the physician prefaces his remarks with the use of the patient's first name.

Thus, the first patient of the morning warranted an elaborated apology, along with title and surname as the terms of address. The second patient elicited an announcement and explanation, but no term of address. The third patient evoked a brief apology, and a first-name salutation. Over the course of this physician's interactions with three consecutive patients, we find distinctive differences in his greeting behaviors. The "punchline" is: The first patient that morning was a white male, 36 years of age; the second patient was a white female, 32 years of age; and the third, a Black male, 36 years of age. With differences in the race and gender of his objects of address, this doctor used substantially different greetings and salutations.[13]

To be sure, an N of one is merely that. Since no other physicians in this collection were recorded across a number of exchanges with different patients, this "finding" might be described as merely an anecdote within the confines of a strictly quantitative analysis. However, the richness of detail evidenced in this single physician's behaviors indicate that further research may uncover considerable variation in physicians' naming practices, depending on patients' identities.

In sum, physicians' uses of address terms for patients also displayed patterned regularities. First names were used far more often than formal terms, but the use of either was confined to particular local contexts. Physicians, like patients, employed terms of address to summon patients' attention to particular utterances. But the most common use of address terms for doctors was the issuance of greetings or farewells. While patients remained "anonymous" through most of physicians' interactions with them, they were addressed directly in the course of opening up or closing down states of talk.

Sociable Conversation in Medical Discourse

Recall Korsch and Negrete's (1972) finding that in pediatric exchanges, physicians' communications with mothers conveyed little "positive affect." In their data, joking matters, salutations, and the use of patients' names were infrequent occurrences, despite the fact that the implementation of such civilities generally produced favorable outcomes. Although the analysis presented in this chapter addressed laughter in particular (rather than joking matters in general), we can note parallels between Korsch and Negrete's results and those reported here.

To the extent that laughter can be seen as an index of "sociable" conversation, physicians and patients in this collection (as in theirs) indulged in very little of it.[14] Moreover, that which they *did* indulge in was marked by an asymmetric distribution between doctors and patients. Patients invited laughter far more frequently than doctors, but their laughter invitations stood a much lesser chance of acceptance. Thus, patients appear to be relatively disadvantaged in initiating this form of social exchange. This finding directly contradicts a suggestion found in Coser's (1960) review of existing research on the subject; namely, "in laughter, all are equal; social barriers, such as those of status, temporarily are lowered" (p. 81). Instead, we find a distribution of laughter that follows the status hierarchy between physicians and patients: It is the doctor who laughs last.[15]

Patterned asymmetries were also evident in the terms of address used by doctors and patients in this collection. In the third of exchanges containing any form of address, doctors employed familiar terms that patients did not return. Moreover, no physician was ever addressed by first name in the 532 pages of transcript. In general, then, naming practices in these medical encounters offer support for Goffman's (1967) hypotheses: "Between status equals we may expect to find interaction guided by symmetrical familiarity. Between superordinate and subordinate we may expect to find asymmetrical relations, with the superordinate having the right to exercise certain familiarities which the subordinate is not allowed to reciprocate" (p. 64).

However, two findings in particular warrant further investigation. First, the physicians and patients in this corpus of materials generally *avoided* using terms of address while interacting with one another. Such reciprocal non-usage would not have been predicted by Korsch and Negrete's (1972) analysis, nor by conventional sociolinguistic approaches to the meaning of address terms. For example, Bosmajian (drawing on Saroyn, 1953) suggests that "To be unnamed is to be unknown, to have no identity" (1974:2). This perspective equates receipt of a name with attainment of a human state, and hence, the absence of a name as a negation of an individual's humanity. But this approach also takes the non-naming of certain entities as a sign of reverence. It views taboo names, like taboo words in general, as signifying the profound respect accorded their potency (Bosmajian, 1974:3–5; Frazer, 1951:302; Trudgill, 1974:29–32). Testimony to the power of gods, priests, and other high church officials is revealed by the reluctance of mere mortals to utter their names.

Obviously, we cannot have it both ways. Whatever the physician's "state of grace" vis-à-vis the patient, the *reciprocal* dispreference for address terms in these data recommends alternative explanation. One possibility resides in the fact that the physician-patient exchange is a dyadic encounter, in which turn-taking between speakers presents only two conceivable choices: Either the physician or the patient will be the "next" speaker after completion of any given turn. One need for address terms (to select a next speaker following completion of a current speaker's turn) is made less urgent in dyadic interchanges (see Sacks et al., 1974), and we would expect fewer address terms would be used in them than in multi-party encounters.

It is also possible that avoidance of address terms may avert explicit acknowledgment of status differences between parties to an exchange. Given that the use of address terms can display the nature of status relationships, avoidance of such usage may well serve to obviate acknowledgment of those relationships. Where status differences are involved, the absence of address terms may coat encounters with a thin veneer—of unacknowledged inequality. Conversely, the repetition of asymmetric forms of address may cement what may only have been implicit prior to their use.

The issue, in any event, cannot be resolved outside the contexts in which these things occur. It is not simply the presence or absence of terms of address, but also whether their forms are used symmetrically or asymmetrically by parties involved (Goffman, 1967). To observe that doctors rarely use patients' names is to see only one side of the picture. The import of this observation cannot be established without looking at how often patients use doctors' names—and how often they avoid using any names at all.[16]

A second matter calling for further study pertains to the local context of interaction in which address terms were employed between physicians and patients in this collection. For example, these encounters evidenced one-way introductions between parties to talk, with physicians presenting themselves by title plus surname, while patients initiated no self-introductions. Physicians' use of titles and surnames in introducing themselves may, of course, be related to patients' subsequent tendencies to address them formally. However, they may also be related to patients' lack of self-introductions. Where patients are "second parties" to initiate these civilities (e.g., where they are waiting to see the doctor), preferences expressed by their co-participants' introductions have considerable import for subsequent talk. Hence, physicians who open up states of talk by introducing themselves in formal terms may unwittingly present patients with a dilemma: Whether to use their own titles and surnames in return (and risk being seen as disrespectful) or employ their first names (and potentially display themselves as lower-status persons in their relationships with doctors). Rather than either of these alternatives, patients in this collection used no names at all.

Beyond first encounters between persons, greetings are generally used to cement (or alter) social relationships and open up states of talk (cf. Frankel and Beckman, 1981). Coupled with the information provided in past exchanges, greetings can upgrade or downgrade the basis for familiarity in an encounter here and now: "When a person begins a mediated or immediate encounter, he already stands in some kind of social relationship to the others concerned, and expects to stand in a given relationship to them after the particular encounter ends. . . . Greetings provide a way of showing that relationship is still what it was at the termination of the previous coparticipation . . ." (Goffman, 1967:41). Among physicians and patients in this collection, the use of address terms in greetings was clearly a physician-initiated phenomenon. Only one patient (the 56 year old who was mentally retarded) ever responded to a physician salutation by using the doctor's name. Given that most patients were first-named by physicians who greeted them, it is perhaps no surprise that their responses to doctors' salutations did not include doctors' names. If physicians introduce themselves by title and surname but address their patients familiarly, patients may have little choice but to accept physicians' definitions of the situation or avoid naming (i.e., defining) altogether.

To be sure, the analysis of naming practices in these data rests on detailed inspection of a small corpus of preliminary materials. Considered individually, none of these findings amounts to much. Whether physicians greet their patients by first names (or not at all) might be regarded as not particularly relevant to the health care of patients or their satisfaction with those who provide it. And, whether or not physicians employ their titles as well as their surnames in introducing themselves to patients, they are still doctors, after all (cf. Goffman, 1979:6). However, the minute subtleties conveyed by such practices and their implications for ongoing interaction are far from trivial. Introductions, for example, can serve as alignment strategies, orienting their users to the terms involved in particular exchanges. Greetings, as Goffman notes, "serve to clarify and fix the roles that participants will take during the occasion of talk and to commit participants to these roles" (1967:4). Thus, the substance of these small ceremonies, involving perhaps only a few seconds of interchange, can have considerable impact on the course of subsequent interaction between participants.

Finally, to the extent that joking remarks, salutations, and the use of parties' names help to constitute an unequal relationship between doctor and patient, these "preliminaries" may impede other attempts to facilitate two-way communication in medical encounters. As we have seen, the organization of such civilities appears to be remarkably context-sensitive (e.g., varying the greeting behavior of one physician with differences in the race and gender of his patients). At the very least, then, these findings suggest a danger in excluding "miscellaneous, or social comments" from research on physician-patient communication.

To be sure, much of the study of relations between physician and patient is predicated on the assumption of interactional asymmetry. Hence, if analysts assume, a priori, that doctors' abilities to provide medical care are contingent on their interactional control over patients, sociable commentary between the two may seem a residual, even trivial, concern. However, many analysts have also treated physician-patient interaction as a *byproduct* of the doctor-patient relationship—rather than as a means of constituting the relationship itself.

CHAPTER 8

Conclusions

> A fairly standard and not unreasonable response to a detailed sociological description of some small segment of the world is "so what?" Description can become an end in itself, and, in so far as there is any pleasure in the rigours of analysis and writing, most of the joy comes from making one small piece fit with another and tidying up all the loose ends. . . . These obsessions are rarely shared by readers, who are more concerned with the point of the whole enterprise. (Strong, 1979:183)

At this point in any book, one is sorely tempted to tie up the loose ends in a solid, unbreakable knot. For writers of fiction, the task is perhaps easiest: sorting out the heroes and villains, dispatching remaining characters to their destinies, or, perhaps, finally revealing "who done it." For narrators of nonfictional accounts, the job is somewhat more difficult, but aided, certainly, by what turn out to be "the facts of the matter," if only retroactively. For reporters such as this one (who might be seen to fall somewhere between these extremes), the work is harder still: arriving at carefully grounded generalizations, acknowledging their limitations, and drawing implications from them . . . all the while stricken by a fundamental "sociological urge to explain the world in a swift paragraph" (Strong, 1979:183). In stories like mine, there are no heroes or villains, and "the facts of the matter" do not lend themselves to tidy knots.

Thus, this last chapter is not a neat one. Here, I attempt a synthesis of my findings on encounters between doctors and patients in order to assess their significance for the study of physician-patient interaction in general. Of necessity, this task entails a review of what we have learned so far and—equally important—of what remains as mere speculation.

ASSESSING ASYMMETRY: A SUMMARY VIEW

In the face of growing concern over problems associated with doctor-patient communication, social science has offered few solutions. As we saw in Chapters 1 and 2, research in the field has by and large restricted itself to theoretical accounts of the physician-patient relationship and sundry empirical investigations of patient compliance, patient satisfaction, and physician control. Neither of these approaches has taken communication between doctors and patients as a topic unto itself.

Theoretical accounts have been heavily influenced by Parsons (1951; 1975), who emphasized the essential asymmetry of therapeutic relationships. In Parsons's view, communication between patients and their doctors is largely prestructured by institutionalized expectations regarding their behaviors (e.g., affective neutrality for physicians and situational dependency for patients). Although critics of this model have been many, none has refuted Parsons's initial premise; namely, that doctors' abilities to provide medical care depend on their control over patients.

Yet this assumption has gone untested. Theories of the physician-patient relationship have failed to explain how physician control is established and they have suggested few empirical guidelines for assessing its effects. In general, such works have tended to reduce a dynamic process of interaction between people to a "script" between well-rehearsed actors.

Assorted empirical studies have echoed the asymmetric theme, without providing verifiable evidence to support it.[1] Often, this lack is an artifact of applied research interests. For example, studies of compliance have used various features of verbal interaction to explore conditions under which patients will obey doctors' orders. In like fashion, investigations of patient satisfaction have treated interaction as a resource rather than as a topic of research. Further, many empirical studies of physician control have in fact excluded social interaction from their research designs, concentrating instead on doctors' and patients' perceptions of communication with one another.[2]

This book began with the suggestion that the study of interaction between practitioners and patients is not substantially advanced by purely theoretical accounts of asymmetries between them. Rather, I proposed that it should start with the systematic examination of talk itself through which physician-patient relationships are established and maintained. Hence, my analyses focused on the social organization of discourse between physicians and patients in an actual medical setting, considering in detail such matters as turn-taking, question-answer sequencing, resolutions of misunderstandings, and the exchange of sociable commentary.

Employing Sacks et al.'s (1974) model of turn-taking in conversation, I established a theoretical basis for distinguishing interruptions (or violations of speaker turns) from other types of simultaneous speech events, such as errors in transition timing between turns or displays of independent knowledge. With this framework, I attempted to examine the empirical bases for such claims as Parsons's regarding the essential asymmetry of the doctor-patient relationship.

In Chapter 4, we learned that encounters between patients and male physicians lent support to the asymmetrical model: Male physicians interrupted their patients (especially their Black patients) far more often than the reverse, and they appeared to use interruptions to exercise control in their interactions with patients. However, there was no evidence which indicated that this pattern of physician-initiated interruption was beneficial for patients' health. If anything, the exercise of this form of control seemed likely to hinder doctors' efforts at healing, through the loss of valuable information pertaining to patient treatment. Moreover, for exchanges involving female physicians, the asymmetrical relationship was exactly reversed: Patients interrupted their female physicians as much or more than their doctors interrupted them. Thus, patterns of interactions between patients and women doctors conflict with Parsons's description of the general pattern.

The number of female physicians included in this collection was very small, although perhaps proportionate to the number of women in medicine. However, growing numbers of women in medical schools and increased concerns for their impact (as women in "a man's world") suggest that patients' interactions with female physicians constitute an important topic for further study. Theoretical accounts of the physician-patient relationship (which tend to view communication as an "exchange of information") have not only failed to acknowledge that people comprise information networks, but have also ignored such fundamental components of human identity as gender as relevant variables in the exchange (see also West, 1982). For findings reported here, it appears that gender may have primary salience over status where women physicians are concerned. These data suggest that gender may account to a "master" status (Hughes, 1945), even where other power relations are involved.

Information exchange per se was the point of departure for the analysis of questions and answers in Chapter 5. There, I observed that doctor-patient interaction would seem to offer an especially important opportunity for an exchange of information, since its presence or absence in this context might have life-and-death implications. However, the examination of actual medical encounters indicates that questions and answers do not operate to effect a two-way flow of information between patients and their doctors. Physicians initiated the overwhelming majority of the total questions observed, while patients tended to stutter when they posed their infrequent queries to doctors.

To be sure, some patients were involved with physicians they had known for three years at the time of recording, while others were meeting physicians for the first time. Some visits were occasioned by long-standing problems, while others were prompted by discoveries of new symptoms. In spite of these variations, exchanges in this collection displayed a systematic and asymmetric pattern. Quantitative and qualitative evidence suggests that physicians stand in nearly god-like relation to their patients—as entities "not to be questioned."

Whatever their state of grace, though, doctors also risk losing a great deal when mishearings and misunderstandings pass unnoticed in their interactions with patients. For medical encounters, a lack of mutual intelligibility between speakers can have major repercussions (e.g., mis-diagnosis, mis-treatment, and even charges of malpractice). So, it seemed reasonable to hypothesize that some alternative to direct questions might be available to ensure that physicians and patients are heard and understood by one another.

Such an alternative appeared in doctors' and patients' use of question-like items that did not function to elicit "answers" per se. These interrogative forms, often treated as residual to the "real" work of information exchange, are primary means available to speakers for establishing ongoing hearing and understanding of speech itself. Included in the analysis in Chapter 6 were requests for repair of prior utterances, requests for confirmation of prior utterances, and markers of surprise at prior utterances.

While patient-initiated questions were strongly dispreferred in these encounters, patients' conditionally relevant question-types were not. We saw that such queries were initiated less frequently than questions, but when they appeared, they displayed virtually symmetrical distributions between doctors and patients. Hence, they seem to offer an alternative, mutually accessible means of establishing understanding between parties to talk.

Like medical misunderstandings, laughter and sociable commentary have routinely been excluded from previous studies of doctor-patient communication. The social cement of friendly chitchat (e.g., laughter, salutations, and the mutual exchange of names) has often been dismissed as "miscellaneous" or "preliminary to" the real business at hand. But findings reported in Chapter 7 add some interesting dimensions to our knowledge of the nature of the relationship between patients and their doctors. For example, if laughter can be seen as an index of sociable conversation, it appears that participants in medical encounters indulge in very little of it. Moreover, that which they do indulge in exhibits an asymmetric distribution between physicians and patients. Patients in these exchanges invited laughter far more often than doctors, but their laughter invitations had a much lesser likelihood of acceptance. Thus, conventional perspectives on laughter, which view it as a means of dissolving social barriers, do not appear to have much utility in medical encounters. Rather, it seems that the organization of laughter follows the status hierarchy between physicians and patients: It is the doctor who laughs last.

Terms of address also exhibited asymmetrical distributions between physicians and patients in this collection. Patients addressed physicians using formal terms exclusively, but physicians tended to use first names in addressing their patients, particularly when those patients were Black. Generally, naming practices followed the principle of symmetry between equals and asymmetry between dominants and subordinates.

In their entirety, the results of this research suggest a rich but complex model of physician-patient interaction. As we have seen, some aspects of medical discourse do indeed exhibit the sorts of organization one would expect on the basis of previous theoretical accounts of the doctor-patient relationship. In general, physicians were the ones who asked the questions, interrupted their co-parties to talk, and initiated the familiarities in these encounters. Conversely, patients generally were the question answerers, the recipients of interruption, and the ones to use formal terms of address in naming their co-participants.

However, this asymmetric script is far from a complete portrayal of what we have learned. For example, patients interrupted women doctors more than the reverse; the organization of conditionally relevant queries exhibited a symmetrical distribution between parties to talk; and for doctors and patients alike, terms of address were the exception rather than the rule. Thus, theories of the physician-patient relationship that attribute unilateral control of interaction to physicians do not find total support in these data. Recall Wolinsky's (1980) summation on Parsons's perspective of the matter: "In everyday and *especially* health related interaction, the practitioner commands and receives deference from others, allowing the practitioner to dominate interpersonal encounters" (p. 164). In retrospect, this description seems vastly oversimplified; as we have seen, "dominance" in these medical encounters was interactionally constituted between parties to talk. Rather than a script between well-rehearsed actors, the interaction between doctor and patient appears to emerge as an ever-unfolding drama, the final scenes of which are always subject to improvisation (e.g., when the doctor is a "lady").

To be sure, if our interest in "interactional control" is restricted to selected features of face-to-face encounters (e.g., question asking, interrupting, or initiating familiarities), the asymmetrical model seems robust enough. And such restrictions have frequently been imposed by applied empirical studies of physician-patient communication (such as investigations of patient compliance or satisfaction). But a focus on talk as a resource for achieving certain goals has yielded the same reliance on untested hypotheses regarding the doctor-patient relationship; namely, that physicians' abilities to provide medical care depend on their interactional control over patients. If institutionalized asymmetry were a requisite component of all therapeutic relations, one would expect to find it manifested in every encounter between those who heal and those who come to them for treatment. Yet, as we have seen, not only are certain categories of doctors (e.g., women physicians) and patients (e.g., male patients) excepted from general rules regarding asymmetry (e.g., that doctors interrupt patients more often than the reverse), but general rules simply have no application for other aspects of interaction (e.g., the organization of conditionally relevant queries or the reciprocal dispreference for address terms in physician-patient talk).

At this point, I must remind readers of the limitations of this research. As I noted earlier, these interactions occurred in the context of only a single kind of physician-patient contact—primary care. Moreover, the visits in which these interactions were recorded all involved ambulatory patients (rather than invalids or hospitalized patients). Finally, these naturally occurring exchanges comprise neither a standardized nor random sample. Therefore, projections from these findings to descriptions of physicians, patients, or medical encounters in general cannot be justified.

What I do take to be generalizable are the routine interactional problems that are posed for physicians and patients whenever they come face to face with one another: maintaining an orderly exchange of turns at talk, regulating a flow of information, resolving potential misunderstandings, and engaging in social amenities (e.g., greetings, introductions, and the mutual exchange of names). Detailed inspection of these medical encounters suggests that physicians and patients resolve such interactional problems in orderly and patterned ways.

I turn now to a consideration of the potential implications of these patterns for our understanding of the physician-patient relationship.

What is a Medical Interview?

I began this work by noting that a "special" (albeit unspecified) sort of communication is generally assumed to characterize the doctor-patient relationship. Journals on medical management have reflected this assumption through voluminous reports of new methods of achieving rapport with patients, tactics for encouraging patients' expression of concerns, and strategies for ensuring that doctors' instructions are heard and understood. Popular magazines have also reflected this assumption in offering practical advice to patients (e.g., how to ask the "right" questions or how to listen to physicians' instructions). I contended that a weakness in all these suggestions pertained to the lack of systematic empirical research on physician-patient communication as a topic in its own right.

Detailed examination of these medical encounters suggests that the production of medical "interviews" (i.e., states of talk in which one party asks questions and the other party answers them or one party's rights to speak carry more weight than another's) is a thoroughly interactional accomplishment. Such an ordering of talk is not merely an outcome of physicians' "dominance" or patients' "passivity." For example, the structural dispreference for patient-initiated questions in these data was jointly produced between physicians and patients in the course of their interaction with one another. Not only did physicians pose questions that restricted their patients' options for answers, but patients themselves stuttered when posing questions to their doctors. Thus, as Frankel (in press b) notes, such matters as control and responsibility in the physician-patient relationship are not readily confined to analytical categorization as attributes of individuals (e.g., heroes or villains). Both doctors and patients are implicated in this social construction of reality.

Thus, traditional sociological formulations of the physician-patient relationship appear to have neglected one of the most important aspects of communication: its essential nature as a social process, with dynamics of its own. In focusing, for example, on characteristics of patients (e.g., educational levels) or characteristics of physicians (e.g., authoritarian tendencies), empirical research has neglected the organization of interaction itself. Further, in explicating expectations attendant to the role of physician (e.g., situational authority) or the role of patient (e.g., situational dependency), theoretical formulations have largely ignored the question of how such roles are implemented in situated interactions between physicians and patients.

At this juncture, I would like to consider some of the practical implications of the research reported here. Although the work is not intended as an alternative "Guide to Understanding Your Doctor" (or—equally important—"Guide to Understanding Your Patient"), it offers a systematic approach for launching future works by those titles. For example, previous empirical studies have yielded at least three general solutions to problems associated with physician-patient communication: (1) eliminate medical jargon, (2) cultivate sociable conversation between physicians and patients, and (3) expand the length of sessions to permit patients' expressions of their chief concerns. But until now, the realization of these goals has been difficult, since little consensus has been obtained on "objective" definitions of their terms. Thus, programs directed toward the deletion of arcane medical terminology from physicians' vocabularies must first know what words constitute jargon to patients. Similarly, doctors striving for friendly rapport with patients require some preliminary information on how their greetings and introductions may communicate sociability rather than social distance. Finally, physicians trying to increase patients' satisfaction with visits by spending more time with them need to know first about the relationship between the quantity and quality of time spent in physician-patient interaction.

Conversation analysis, the framework employed throughout this work, affords a new perspective on these matters.[3] From a methodological standpoint, it permits a means of identifying interactional troubles in the course of their actual production. So, rather than relying on retroactive quizzes to determine which of physicians' instructions or patients' concerns have been heard and understood, we can attend to the *in situ* responses to these speech activities at the time they actually occur. And, where friendly rapport is problematic, we can explore the ways in which the temporal organization of greetings and introductions creates potential dilemmas for participants to talk. Moreover, before unilaterally increasing the amount of time allotted to each medical encounter, physicians and patients can be sensitized to the ways in which their talk structures the quality of whatever time slot is available to them (e.g., through systematic interruption or the chaining of questions in a series).

The emphasis of this form of analysis on the structure of interaction, rather than on the identities of interactional participants, further promises a more humane approach to solving problems of physician-patient communication (see also Frankel [1982a; 1982b; 1983; 1984; in press; in preparation] and Heath [1981; 1982a; 1982b; in press; forthcoming]). Popular stereotypes of "omnipotent" physicians and "helpless" patients have tended to locate responsibility for communicative troubles with individuals themselves and the "kinds of people" the stereotypes depict. Hence, popular accounts of these problems frequently conclude with the suggestion that a "better type" of individual must be recruited for medical training, or a "more sophisticated" patient must be cultivated through extensive education programs. In the interim, patients are urged to "be more assertive," while physicians are encouraged to "be more reflective" in prodding for patients' concerns. Results of my research indicate that both suggestions are likely to be unsuccessful in altering the structural organization of interaction in medical dialogues. For example, "being more assertive" is usually defined as asking more questions of one's physician. But the patient in this collection who posed most questions to her doctor received proportionately fewest answers. Thus, I note that the organizational dispreference for patient-initiated questions may be reflected by physicians' reluctance to answer "too many" of them. With regard to direct questions, then, the assertive patient may suffer more than her less insistent counterparts.

However, focusing on the structure of interaction does not preclude the possibility of transforming situated occasions of face-to-face exchange. At this microanalytic level, structural constraints have a rather different meaning than in macrosociological explanations. Because individual persons comprise the participants in face-to-face interaction, the systems for organizing their exchanges with one another (for taking turns at talk, for effecting repairs of problematic utterances, etc.) remain to be activated in concrete situations. While the systems themselves operate according to a context-free set of principles (e.g., the organization of adjacency pairs dictates that answers follow questions in time and sequential position), they are context-sensitive in their use (e.g., a request for repair may be warranted between a question and its answer). Moreover, the "decision" to implement many of these systems rests with the participants themselves.[4] So, for example, I suggest that conditionally relevant queries might serve as substitutes for some questions in physician-patient dialogues. Given that questions exhibit an asymmetric organization between physicians and patients, if conditionally relevant queries (such as requests for confirmation) were used as replacements for many physician-initiated questions, the resulting organization of medical discourse might assume less interrogational (and more symmetrical) proportions. Rather than constructing medical "interviews," doctors and patients might use these devices to create a structure of talk that allows them further possibilities for a two-way flow of information.

STATUTES AND LIMITATIONS

My remarks are not meant to imply that physicians and patients "choose" such patterns of interaction as we have observed in the absence of external constraints. For example, time is an important dimension of any medical exchange (cf. Schwarz, 1974; Henley, 1977:43–54). Unlike many naturally occurring conversations, encounters between physicians and patients ordinarily transpire within the boundaries of designated time slots (which are themselves set up in advance). Whether such encounters ensue as part of morning rounds in a hospital or afternoon appointments in a clinic, physicians' visits with patients are oriented to the larger temporal structure of clinical practice. While some doctors may allocate more time per patient than others, none is free to conduct routine patient visits in a manner that is oblivious to the constraints of the day's appointments (hence, we find one basis for the special status of "emergency" visits). Like other instances of social exchange that are subject to demands of the clock (e.g., classroom interactions, courtroom interactions, or talk show interactions), the outside boundaries of particular medical exchanges are largely constrained by the contexts in which they occur.

The organization of instrumental medical tasks poses further limitations on the organization of interaction in medical dialogues. To the extent that patients' expressions of their concerns constitute a necessary precondition for physicians' formulations of diagnoses and instructions, the sequential ordering of these tasks forms a backdrop for interactional activities. Thus, physician recipients of patients' "delayed complaints" must recycle their own agendas for action if such complaints are to be managed in the course of visits in progress.

However, I do mean to recommend that we re-examine our empirical bases for attributing observed communication patterns between physicians and patients to factors beyond their control. For example, diagnosis is commonly viewed as a process of hypothesis-testing (i.e., subjecting an ordered set of theories to an ordered set of proof procedures). From this perspective, doctors conversing with patients are seen to be simultaneously engaged in processing information regarding their patients' health. Hence, since information-processing is conducted deductively, a patient's question or addition of something "more" than is called for by the doctor may be seen as interrupting the doctor's cognitive deductions. However, this perspective also assumes that the process of diagnosis is externally imposed and transpires entirely within the physician's head, rather than evolving between doctor and patient in the course of their interaction with one another.[5]

Similarly, the review of systems (respiratory, circulatory, gastrointestinal, etc.) is often cited as an external factor which influences the course of communication between physician and patient. In the process of such a review, physicians impose a sort of checklist which is thought to cover all points in the system. In so doing, they do not search for "new" information, but for checks on "old" information already encoded in patients' records (e.g., "You having any shortness of breath?", "Pain in the chest?", or "Heart palpitations?"). Once the review is in process, a patient's introduction of a question or additional material not called for (e.g., "By the way, doctor") can disrupt the entire structure of the checklist.

But nowhere is it written that the review of systems must be conducted to ensure an adequate flow of information to physician from patient. Indeed, one physician-friend has dispensed with this process entirely, finding that all but the most problematic cases will unfold naturally—and in the patient's own words—in response to something as simple as "What brings you here today?" By encouraging the patient's expression of concerns in holistic fashion, she not only saves time (e.g., avoiding rote questions about irrelevant aspects of the patient's health),[6] but circumvents patients' introduction of "delayed" complaints. As we learned in Chapters 5 and 6, when patients' speech is restricted to answering doctors' questions, they may find few chances to pose questions of their own. But when patients' speech is employed to produce jointly ratified plans, explanations and courses of future action with their doctors, both doctor and patient may find opportunities to resolve potential troubles in talk before they represent threats to the physician-patient relationship.

My notion here is that some might attribute results of this investigation to similar constraints external to the talk that goes on between doctor and patient. Popular and scholarly sources alike have cited patients' "ignorance" and physicians' "dominance" as two of the most compelling factors in explaining gaps in doctor-patient communication. But at this point in our knowledge, such "explanations" do not have the status of reasons, but of hypotheses, requiring further explanation. Moreover, on the basis of findings reported here, I would caution against taking selected patterns of interaction as indices of differential knowledge structures or differential institutionalized expectations, when an alternative analysis can be grounded in the organization of interaction itself (see Schegloff, 1980:146).

The Everyday World as a Phenomenon[7]

If face-to-face interaction is a primary arena for the social construction of human relations, interactions between physicians and patients would seem to offer an especially important analytical opportunity for understanding the dynamics of social inequality. "Patients" are people from all walks of life. They are black and white, women and men, and poor as well as affluent. "Physicians," on the other hand, are normatively white, male, and upper middle class. Moreover, they are practitioners of one of the most prestigious and lucrative occupations in this country.[8] Thus, occasions of encounters between doctors and patients afford a wealth of potential insights into micropolitical aspects of face-to-face interaction.

The rationale for my research was obtained from the assumption that our social world is in large part constructed of and through our mundane exchanges with one another. We inhabit a variety of situated identities, of course: as parents and children, men and women, teachers and students, or physicians and patients. The findings of this research offer us better understanding of how these identities are accomplished in everyday life.

Conventionally, social inequality is taken to mean unequal access to life resources—in the occupational structure, the family division of labor, and other institutional contexts where life chances are determined. As Henley (1977) observes: "Most discussions of power deal with broad scenarios, the power distribution within communities, the nation, the world. They are apt to be written by political scientists, and focus on control of wealth, industries, political bodies, and armies" (p. 20). Hence, the mortar of social stratification is generally conceptualized in terms of goods, services, and material relations between social classes.

However, face-to-face relations between human beings are no less stratified by more subtle sorts of mortars. Such experiences as being interrupted while speaking, finding it difficult to "get a word in edgewise," or suspecting that one's conversational partner is not in fact listening are products of micropolitical dynamics in social exchange. Whereas wealth and material possessions testify to our positions within the institutionalized hierarchy, "The human tendency to use signs and symbols means that evidence of social worth and of mutual evaluations will be conveyed by very minor things . . . An unguarded glance, a momentary change in tone of voice, an ecological position taken or not taken can drench talk with judgmental significance" (Goffman 1967:33). Goffman's remarks underscore the importance of detailed empirical studies of situated social interactions for our understanding of social inequality as an experienced phenomenon. Through what actual behaviors are the social roles of physician and patient acted out on given occasions that they encounter one another? How are medical definitions of situations superimposed over lay definitions in the course of the organization of doctors' and patients' talk with one another? And, perhaps most important, how do power and control achieve salience across a range of human interactions and a variety of human identities? These are the substantive problems this work has sought to address.

But such problems are implicated in the variety of interactions that comprise our existing social relations with one another. Social roles always remain to be enacted in particular situations; professional definitions of situations rarely agree with lay definitions; and power and control constitute enduring problems of social life. Thus, detailed analysis of the situated elements of discourse affords us a fresh perspective on the problem of social order *as embodied in* face-to-face interaction between people.

Notes

Chapter 1   Troubles with Talk Between Doctors and Patients

1. Apparently, when written discourse is involved, this gap is not limited to physicians' communications with patients. A survey conducted by the *American Druggist* (May 1983) reports that 50 percent of pharmacists have dispensed the wrong medication to patients due to illegible handwriting on physicians' prescriptions.

2. A summary of this conference, *Women's Leadership and Authority in the Health Professions: Proceedings of a Conference at UC Santa Cruz, June 19-21, 1977*, is available from the Program for Women in Health Services, University of California, San Francisco (mimeo).

3. For example, women constituted less than 9 percent of graduates from U.S. medical schools in 1972–1973 (Braslow and Heins, 1981). Moreover, though they comprised 23 percent of graduating doctors by 1978–1979, over half of them were concentrated in specialties with lowest earnings: Pediatrics, 19 percent; General Practice, 17 percent; Psychiatry, 16 percent; and Family Practice, 6 percent (Mattera, 1980).

4. Although much work in this area focuses on spoken interaction, the approach has advanced our understanding of nonverbal behavior as well (see Frankel, 1983; C. Goodwin, 1980; 1981; M. H. Goodwin, 1980; and Heath, 1981; in press, for excellent examples).

5. There are 21 dyadic interactions included in the data base. Of these, three involve the same physician in encounters with different patients, and two involve the same patient in encounters with different physicians.

6. By "progressive," I mean oriented to patient care in a social context (see Chapter 3 for a more detailed description of the special characteristics of this medical specialty).

7. These are also technical problems for conversationalists in general. One aim of this work is to illuminate the ways in which doctor-patient encounters differ from other conversational exchanges; another aim is to assess the features they share in common.

8. An alternative approach to organizing these chapters might draw on the organization of instrumental activities contained in medical interviews. However, existent accounts of the organization of these activities (e.g., medical history-taking, physical examination, diagnosis, etc.) tend to presuppose the primacy of instrumental tasks over interactional ones, without questioning the interdependence of the two (see Chapter 5).

Chapter 2   The Study of Doctor-Patient Communication

1. To be sure, Freidson (1961) might also be read as questioning the bases for patients' passivity. In suggesting that the physician-patient relationship entails a clash of perspectives (between the professional's world of

medicine and the patient's lay referral system), he does imply that medical encounters constitute occasions for negotiated conflict. However, Freidson does not debate the "technical specificity" of the physician's role (Bloom and Wilson, 1979:288). Moreover, he agrees that physicians' authority over patients is largely conferred by institutional means: *"What distinguishes the professional from all other consulting experts is his capacity to solve some of these problems of authority by formal institutionalized means. His solution minimizes the role of persuasive evidence in his interaction with his clientele"* (Freidson, 1970a:110; italics in original).

2. Such studies are conducted by a hybrid group of medical researchers, social scientists, and public health physicians.

3. Differences between Korsch and Negrete's (1972) and McKinlay's (1975) findings also may have resulted from the different populations they studied. McKinlay's data were collected in Scotland; Korsch and Negrete's data were assembled in the United States.

4. The problem here is a fundamental one in the sociology of knowledge: How does one know what someone else might not know? Shapiro (1978) offers a delightful account of the physician's acquisition of technical jargon in the course of basic medical training: "During an early meeting of my medical class in first year, we were promised a five thousand word increase in our vocabularies within the year. Learning those words turned out to be a tedious process and unhappily, many of them were of little use later on in our studies and in medical practice" (p. 164). Of course, by the time members of Shapiro's class "hit the wards" in the last years of medical school, they were fluent in this "second language." However, by that time, they had also forgotten which items of their new lexicons seemed arcane or esoteric on first encounter.

5. Some analyses of discourse also rely on this conceptualization (e.g., Fisher, 1983; Shuy, 1983; Tannen and Wallat, 1983; and Waitzkin and Stoekle, 1976).

Chapter 3   Methods, Measurement, and Medical Encounters

1. To get some notion of the diversity of American medicine, it is worth noting that twenty-two different medical specialty boards were approved by the American Medical Association in 1973 (American Medical Association, 1973).

2. "Primary care" doctors are physicians who ordinarily make first contact with patients—general practitioners, family physicians, general internists, and general pediatricians (Mechanic, 1979). Specialist and subspecialist practitioners generally see patients on referrals or consultations (initiated by primary care physicians).

3. "Ambulatory" patients are those not confined in bed (e.g., in hospitals or convalescent homes).

4. Moreover, in examining results of the 1980 National Ambulatory Care Survey, Frankel observes: "Even if one takes the cautious stance of disqualifying all instances of serious disease as a criterion . . . an impressive number of patients seeking care, 290,680,000 of an estimated 577,000,000 appear to be 'healthy,' i.e., nonsymptomatic" (1983:22).

5. To be sure, Freidson's (1970b) distinction between "expectations"

and "performance" of the physician's role is pertinent here. The fact that family practice is such a new medical specialty perhaps explains the lack of social scientific research on its practitioners in practice. For example, Mechanic's (1979) review of "Physicians" in the *Handbook of Medical Sociology* had relatively little to say about family physicians: "The internist is seen as an intellectual problem-solver, while the surgeon is seen as more aggressive and active. The family practitioner, in contrast, tends to be less conceptual and more gregarious than the internist" (p. 179). However, personality characteristics of family practitioners and other physicians are inventoried in McCauley (1978).

6. To make a long story short: my ultimate discovery of (and access to) a suitable research setting was a consequence of good luck and a good grapevine. One of the faculty members in this setting had obtained his doctorate from the institution at which I was employed in 1979. He called his alma mater to find out whether any graduate students might be interested in short-term employment there. The faculty member who received his call knew of no graduate students that were looking for such employment. However, he said, "I know a faculty member who'd certainly be interested in what you're doing there!" In this way, I obtained my initial contact with the research site.

Prior to this call, I had taken every conceivable opportunity to let friends and colleagues know what I was looking for. Some, for example, had friends who were physicians in our community; others served on local boards to supervise neighborhood health services. Although none of these contacts proved as ideal for my needs as the one I eventually made, it was the process of making such contacts that finally yielded results. From personal experience, then, I recommend this form of "networking" very highly.

7. For a detailed analysis of the discourse processes involved in securing "informed consent" in such a setting, see Robillard et al., 1983.

8. Two physicians in this collection are not residents. One, an alumnus of the training program, still sees patients at the Center after completing his residency four years ago. The other, a faculty member on the staff, also sees patients there. With regard to the analyses that follow, I found no differences evidenced between these doctors' exchanges with patients and those of resident physicians.

9. The year in which these data were collected (1979), the Center admitted its first Black (male) resident. Unfortunately, he was not recorded during the time these tapes were made.

10. As I noted earlier, these are generic problems of face-to-face interaction rather than specific problems of physician-patient encounters (see Chapter 1, Note 6). At issue here are the ways in which these interactional problems are articulated with (or against) other characteristics of the medical encounter (e.g., the necessity for diagnosis of illness) and other features of the doctor-patient relationship (its essential asymmetry, the inequality of physicians' and patients' knowledge bases, etc.).

11. As noted in Chapter 2, this focus on the systematics of utterance production (or "actual enactment" of talk's telling) also distinguishes conversation analysis from discourse-analytic enterprises (see Schlegloff, 1981:1–4).

12. Thus, canons of evidence further distinguish this mode of inquiry from many discourse analyses (cf. Cicourel, 1975; 1977; 1978; 1981b; Gumperz, 1982:153–171; Labov and Fanshel, 1977:24–27).

Chapter 4   Turn-Taking in Doctor-Patient Dialogues

1. To be sure, computers are expected to play an increasingly important part in the doctor-patient relationship, especially in the taking of medical histories. Thus far, their use appears to be limited to contexts in which information gathering can be reduced to a set of standardized questions and answers (but see Chapter 5 for some of the dangers associated with such query and response patterns).

2. Here, I must emphasize that *overlap* and *interruption* are two general categories, not meant to encompass the range of specific simultaneous speech events that may occur between two or more speakers. More detailed discussion of finer distinctions is provided in West, 1978 (including a 12-page coding scheme for classifying initiations, resolutions, and retrievals of simultaneous speech).

3. Except where otherwise designated, fragments of talk between doctors and patients are excerpted from exchanges in my collection. Dyads are numbered 1 through 21, and line numbers are provided for each fragment.

4. As indicated in Note 3, the categorization of instances of simultaneous speech involved a detailed coding scheme (see West 1978) designed to distinguish violations of speakers' rights (interruptions) from other types of simultaneity (e.g., errors in transition timing, displays of active listening, simultaneous starts, and continuations of prior incomplete turns.) Despite its complexity, the coding scheme yields a high rate of intercoder reliability: in this case, 87 percent agreement between an independent coder and myself. Disagreements (typically, over instances of overlap rather than interruption) were resolved by discussion of the individual utterances in question.

5. An anecdote may help to illuminate this point. A friend of mine has suffered all her life from a chronic but rare lung disorder. Prior to the discovery of sulfa drugs, people died from this disorder; now, it is manageable with routine monitoring and treatment. My friend has traveled around the world, and visited numerous physicians for treatment of her condition. Since her disorder is a rare one, she often discovers that she knows more about her problem than the doctors she goes to for treatment. And yet, she observes that most physicians insist on going through a standard battery of questions and strategies before they begin to treat her complaints seriously. Thus, suggestions she tries to raise concerning useful new ways of coping with her disorder are often aborted by physicians' insistence on a litany of complaints and disorders described in medical textbooks.

6. My use of quotation marks around the term *lady* is meant to highlight this point. Lakoff suggests that this term operates as a euphemism for *woman*: "Just as we do not call whites 'Caucasian-Americans,' there is no felt need to refer to men commonly as 'gentlemen.' And just as there is a need for such terms as 'Afro-Americans,' there is similarly felt a need for 'lady.' One might even say that when a derogatory epithet exists, a parallel

euphemism is deemed necessary" (1975:21). To the extent that "lady" in fact operates as a euphemism (i.e., rendering the fact of femaleness less distasteful and more respectable than "woman"), its coupling with respected occupational terms (e.g., "lady lawyer," "lady doctor," or "lady engineer") becomes a fascinating object of study for students of folklore.

7. Worth speculation: whether this designation ("our new women residents") would have been used in describing the same people to a male researcher in that setting. Worth noting: Hogan's (1978) contention that the use of personal pronouns in this context implies proprietorship rather than collegial relations.

8. The last portion of this patient's utterance consists of laughter particles ("hungh-hungh-hungh-hungh!"), included in the transcribing conventions (see pp. xiii–xiv).

9. For example, such considerations as limited time and the routinization of medical work may also play a part in physicians' interruptions of patients. However, the time slots allocated to patients in these exchanges are relatively large (thirty minutes per patient) in comparison to the average (see Bains, 1979). Moreover, such factors do not account for the patterns of interruption observed between patients and female physicians.

10. Insofar as "better listening" is related to amount of time spent with patients (see Note 9), there is evidence to this effect. Results of the 1980 National Ambulatory Medical Care Survey indicate that women physicians spend more time with patients than men do: "Female physicians spent some time in face-to-face encounter with virtually all their patients, while 3 percent of visits to male physicians were 'o' minutes; that is, patients were treated by a staff member. Male physicians spent less than 11 minutes in 52 percent of their patient encounters; female physicians spent that amount of time in 33 percent. About 39 percent of visits to female physicians lasted 16 minutes or longer, compared with 18 percent of visits with the same duration to males" (U.S. Department of Health, Education and Welfare, 1983b:2–3).

Chapter 5   Questions and Answers between Doctors and Patients

1. Frankel's (in press b) use of the term "dispreferred" is consistent with the language of conversation analysis. Ordinarily, "preference" is regarded as a matter of personal opinion or individual choice. However, systematic studies of conversation suggest that personal opinions and individual choices may have little to do with some patterned regularities in social interaction between people: "We use the term 'preference' technically to refer not to motivations of the participants, but to sequence- and turn-organizational features of conversation. For example, 'dispreferreds' are structurally delayed in turns and sequences and are (or may be) preceded by other items; dispreferreds may be formed as preferreds" (Schegloff et al., 1977:362).

2. Harvey Sacks first formulated the notion of a "chain rule" for questions in unpublished lectures given at the University of California, Los Angeles, 1966.

3. Goffman (1981b) is misleading here, I think. In reviewing Schegloff and Sacks's (1974) suggestion regarding the indexicality of answers, he contends: "One problem with this view is that in throwing back upon the

asker's question the burden of determining what will qualify as an answer, it implies that what is a question will itself have to be determined in a like manner . . . this formulation leaves no way open for disproof" (Goffman, 1981b:51, n. 35). However, for an unanswered question, "proof" is provided by the relevance of a repetition of the question "or some inference based on the absence of an answer" (Schegloff, 1972:77). Thus, the intelligibility of a question as a question does not rest entirely on the presence of an answer in the next turn space. Of course, as Goffman argues, "When an intended question receives no apparent answer, the asker will often let the matter pass, and so, although there is no phenomenal evidence of a question having been asked, it really has" (personal communication, October 7, 1981). Clearly, such instances are ripe for further empirical study.

4. I use "some equivalent" advisedly here, since my purpose is to suggest an analogy rather than an equivalence. Insofar as any prior utterance serves as a possible repairable, it is impossible to specify the first pair parts of repairables in advance of their occurrences.

5. Thus, head nods and head shakes were included as "answers" when they appeared to be treated that way by parties involved. And questions pertaining to matters other than medical treatment are also included for analysis.

6. In passing, I will note that female patients as a group asked more questions of their doctors than males did: The total number of questions initiated by females was 42 ($\bar{x}$ = 3.8) whereas for males, it was 26 ($\bar{x}$ = 2.6). However, the difference in these aggregate figures is the product of a single "deviant case" (i.e., the 53-year-old white female patient who asked 18 questions of her doctor). With the exclusion of this case, total numbers of questions asked by male and female patients are virtually identical (i.e., 26 and 24).

7. In a study of physicians' communications with children and parents (conducted in the same setting in which my data were collected), Pantell et al. (1982) found that doctors tended to *give* most information to parents but to *collect* most information from children. Thus, children's roles in the doctor-parent-child interactions they studied tended to be those of "answerers" (providers of symptoms and problem-related expressions). While Pantell and his colleagues observed a "progressive involvement of children in substantive communications as they became older" (p. 400), it is possible that adolescents have a hard time shaking their earlier, restricted roles in communications with physicians.

8. Readers may be curious about the incidence of stuttering in questions formulated by physicians. Certainly all doctors' questions did not go off "without a hitch." One exchange between a first-year physician and a patient meeting for the first time displayed more than a few disfluencies in the physician's production of questions. However, the physician exhibited speech disfluencies in the course of formulating many other utterance-types as well. His first visit with the patient, first month in training at the Center and first video monitoring session may have combined to produce more discomfort in his interaction with the patient than would ordinarily have been the case (so he remarked to monitoring faculty members).

By and large, however, physicians' formulations of questions exhibited little evidence of speech disturbances (as can be seen in excerpts presented throughout this chapter).

9. These results also agree with patterns of question-asking observed in discourse-analytic studies (e.g., Fisher, 1983; Paget, 1983; and Todd, 1983). However, as noted in Chapter 2, discourse analyses proceed from a different epistemology from that employed here. Thus, Fisher compares doctors' and patients' uses of questions as devices for displaying "competence"; Paget analyzes the "sequencing and semantic sense of questioning practices"; and Todd is concerned with questions as forms of speech acts (hence, she includes what I see as "conditionally relevant queries" in her analysis of questions per se).

10. An explicit illustration of comparisons between diagnosis and hypothesis-testing is provided by *The Future General Practitioner: Teaching and Learning* (Royal College of General Practitioners, 1972:21–47).

11. Here, I am indebted to Judy Martin, M.D., for her critique of the assumed necessity for "systems reviews" through Yes/No questioning: "It brings to mind Mary Daly's criticism (indictment? exorcism?) of Medicine and Gynecology—one of the characteristics of torture is that it's highly ritualized, to neutralize the horror" (Martin, personal communication, February 24, 1982). Indeed, as Daly (1978) notes: "The therapeutic curers of disorder impose a false order (meaning) upon the histories of their patients/clients. Vying with the unnaturalness of the lithotomy (supine) position, of The Pill, of exogenous estrogens, of cosmetic surgery, this psychically disordering order decomposes and dismembers women's personal histories, recomposing them to match the monotonous beat of the Masters' metronome" (pp. 284–285).

Chapter 6   Medical Misfires: Mishearings, Misgivings, and Misunderstandings

1. Indeed, as Ley (1983) observes, dissatisfaction with information communicated from doctors to patients has not lessened in this time period—even when physicians have been made aware of the problem and have consciously attempted to remedy it.

2. For example, Wallen et al. (1979) transcribed only those portions of tape-recorded dialogues designated as "information-exchange." Their operational definition of information event is as follows: "A request for information (question) or informative statements on a particular topic (explanation). Information events could be distinguished as discrete units because they were separated from one another by pauses or information events produced by another speaker" (p. 138). And whereas Frankel (in press b) does not distinguish "information exchange" from other talk in medical interviews, he views such queries as requests for clarification as " 'normal' troubles." Therefore, they are deliberately excluded from his study of physician-initiated and patient-initiated utterances (p. 12).

3. The authors note that interrogative question terms are not always used to initiate repair of *actual* prior components of another party's speech object. For example:

> Ben: They gotta- a gara̱ge sale.
> Ellen: Where.
> Ben: On Third A̱venoo.

(Schegloff et al., 1977:369, n. 15)

In this fragment, "Where" elicits something more than was present in the utterance preceding it. In my discussion here, I am only interested in initiations of repair directed toward actual prior turn components.

4. "Pardon me?" is not included in Schegloff et al.'s (1977) analysis of devices employed to request repairs. As Jorge Hankamer has pointed out to me, "Pardon me?" operates in a somewhat different way than "Who?" or "What?" with respect to its linguistic implications (e.g., "Where?" might be rebuilt into sentence form as "Where did you go?"). However, from an interactional standpoint, "Pardon me?" does at least the work of requesting repetition of a prior speech object (cf. Austin, 1962). So, I include it in the general category of requests for repair in this analysis.

5. A more detailed discussion of the mechanics involved in such retrospective searches is provided in Schegloff, 1979 (especially pp. 276–280). As Schegloff notes, "A succession of repairs is not organized only by relating any next unit to its prior but that . . . the organization operates for the SERIES AS A WHOLE" (p. 280).

6. This designation originated with Stubbs (1973), who employed it in discourse-analytic fashion to describe the interactional functions of various utterance-types (i.e., the meanings they encoded in talk). Labov and Fanshel (1977) used the term similarly, pointing to the speech acts performed by different classes of requests. My use of "requests for confirmation" diverges from previous usage. Here, I am employing it to refer to the *technical* work performed by these conditionally relevant queries in their local contexts (e.g., eliciting acknowledgment tokens) rather than to their interpretive meanings for individual speakers (see Chapter 2).

7. "Say what?", often used by speakers of Black English, also seems to belong in this class of question-types.

8. Again, "some equivalent" is used deliberately to suggest an analogy rather than an absolute equivalence. If any prior utterance may serve as a possible repairable (Schegloff et al., 1977:363), then it is impossible to specify the first pair parts of repairables in advance of their occurrences (see also Goffman, 1981a:224).

9. This point warrants heavy emphasis for purposes of this analysis. For example, Schegloff and Sacks (1974) observe that items such as "We-ell. . .," "O.K. . .," and "So-ooo"—produced with *downward intonational* contours—can serve as "possible pre-closing" devices to terminate exchanges. Thus, the same lexical item (okay) can provide "a place for new topic beginnings" (p. 246) as well as an opportunity for the other to confirm the intelligibility of a prior utterance.

Further, Frankel (in press) finds "Okay"—with an interrogative pattern—may be used by physicians to solicit "last calls for information" from patients before moving to next activities. However, in the case of solicits, "Okay?" serves as a disjunct marker, which is appended to prior utterances containing bits of evaluation or instruction *after* a discernible gap. Hence, the use of "okay" as a last call for information must *follow* evaluative or instructional comments, but not be immediately appended to them.

Clearly, the subtle distinctions illuminated by these analyses reaffirm the wisdom of painstaking empirical examination and detailed transcribing methodologies.

10. See Ekman and Friesen's (1969) discussion of nonverbal substitutes for verbal rejoinders.

11. This also suggests that the range of "normal troubles" posed by these objects is nearly equally divided between physicians and patients.

12. To be sure, the distribution of requests for repair in these medical encounters is less symmetrical than the other distributions of conditionally relevant queries and warrants further empirical study, e.g., comparing instances of self-correction to other-corrections in data such as these (see Note 13). However, the point to be made here is that in relation to questions per se, requests for repair approximate an equal distribution between physicians and patients.

13. Schegloff et al. (1977) observe that conversations evidence a preference for speakers' repairs of their own prior utterances over repairs initiated by other parties to talk.

14. Interestingly, both instances of physicians' failures to confirm occurred where patients made self-disparaging assertions. In one case, a patient appended a request for confirmation at the end of a series of declarations regarding his lack of discipline and creativity; in the other case, the patient's request for confirmation followed a statement which exaggerated his weight problem. The physicians' reponses thus failed to confirm the intelligibility of patients' self-depreciations.

15. This second suggestion is in fact the major premise of most discourse analyses reviewed in Chapter 2. Here, however, I am concerned with the *technical* production of particular interactional events through speakers' use of specific utterance-types (see Schegloff, 1980: 149–150).

16. Whereas Emerson (1970) found male gynecologists showed a preference for definite articles in reference to women's body parts (e.g., "the vagina" rather than "your vagina"), this excerpt shows a female physician repairing such an instance by substituting a pronoun for a definite article ("in the mou::th- in yer mouth").

17. Goffman suggests that throat clearings constitute "A good example of ritualization: an apparently instrumental act that comes to acquire cummunicative significance" (personal communication, November 30, 1981). For a delightful empirical study of the temporal organization of throat clearings, coughs, sneezes, and sniffs, see Thomas (1980).

18. Data such as these offer further reason to be cautious in attributing observed patterns of discourse (e.g., skewed distributions of questions and answers) to factors external to talk itself (e.g., constraints of hypothesis testing on diagnosis).

19. To be sure, patients' tendencies to produce "delayed complaints" are more often the subject of comments than rigorous empirical study. Although the "By the way" opening is widely recognized among resident physicians in this study, there is reason to believe that its actual incidence is less frequent than it is believed to be (see Robertson, 1981).

Chapter 7   Laughter and Sociable Commentary in Medical Encounters

1. The continued and deliberate exclusion of social amenities from scholarly investigations of medical encounters is perhaps a consequence of an overly task-oriented perspective on these matters. In attending to the instrumental ends of medical discourse (e.g., history taking, examination and diagnosis) researchers may lose sight of the fact that such talk is, first

and foremost, an occasion of face-to-face exchange between human beings (for an important exception, see Emerson [1970] and Note 14, below).

2. To be sure such civilities have been subject to considerable attention outside the confines of social scientific studies. For example, *Ms.* magazine recently published a patient's complaint regarding physicians' overly familiar means of addressing patients. Titled "Hi, Lucille, this is Dr. Gold!" (Natkins, 1983), the article originally appeared in the *Journal of the American Medical Association,* where it prompted a flurry of feedback. Subsequently, comments have appeared in the *Los Angeles Times* (Parachini, 1983), the newsletter of the National Organization for Women *(National NOW Times,* May 1983), *American Medical News* (Bookman, 1984; Mehr, 1984), and the *New England Journal of Medicine* (Conant, 1983). Obviously, the original protest sparked recognition in a wide variety of readers.

3. This "joke's" equivocality rests on two points. First, the physician volunteers laughter before the patient has completed the utterance which would constitute the joke's punchline. While some overlaps in speech seem to effect "displays of recognition" of that which is in the course of being said (Jefferson, 1973), the physician initiates laughter well before the patient's utterance is recognizable or projectable. Second, the patient's *response* to the physician's laughter is similar in form to what Jefferson and Schegloff (1975) term *marked self-retrieval.* Note that the patient drops her utterance midway into its production ("pritty gir:ls walk-"), and then restarts it in the clear ("Pritty gir:ls walk by."). If the utterance was intended as a joke, and had already elicited laughter from its recipient, why would repetition be necessary?

4. Thus, addendums of laughter particles to incomplete utterances did not constitute proper laughter invitations by my operational criteria.

5. The use of "spuriously" here is deliberate. Since this analysis focuses on observed behaviors, it is possible that instances of merely coincidental laughter might be included in the category described as voluntary. For example, the idle daydreams of persons simultaneously engaged in conversation might engender laughter on their part without regard to whatever is in the process of being talked about. Literary sources often refer to such occurrences as instances of "laughing to oneself." However, in face-to-face interaction, participants who "laugh to themselves" are indistinguishable from those who "laugh at others" if they laugh while in the company of those others.

6. The subtitle for this section is borrowed with appreciation from the first chapter of *Words and Women: New Language in New Times* (Miller and Swift, 1976).

7. It is worth noting that the two exchanges exhibiting the classic pattern of asymmetry described by sociolinguists (in which doctors are addressed formally while patients are addressed familiarly) are the same two exchanges that deviated from the general pattern in my earlier analysis of interruptions (see Chapter 4). The two patients involved here (the elderly white female who is hard of hearing and the middle-aged white male who is mentally retarded) may be "exceptional" in more ways than one.

8. In this sense, there may indeed be an asymmetry of knowledge between doctors and patients: not of expert and lay understandings (as discussed in Chapter 2), but of biographical details about the other that are

helpful in orienting introductions. Although patients may also be introduced to doctors in third-party fashion (e.g., by medical assistants, nurse
practitioners, or referring physicians), it is unlikely that they receive the
same breadth of information about physicians as is encoded in their own
medical files (such as birth date, marital status, family history).

9. An alternative explanation might be derived from the nature of
server-client relationships in the work world; namely, servers apparently
are bound to introduce themselves in a variety of contexts in which clients'
names are not expected in return. For example, waiters identify themselves
to restaurant patrons, airline attendants announce themselves to airplane
passengers, and grocery store clerks wear badges offering their identities
to customers in supermarkets. However, in these settings, servers are expected to attend to many clients simultaneously in the co-presence of all of
them. Hence, self-introductions by the servers may merely ensure that no
one client will suffer too long without the servers' attentions. (Would that
merely calling a doctor could provide the same guarantee.)

10. To be sure, most medical clinics (including the Center) employ some
staff members who are not medical doctors (e.g., physicians' assistants,
nurse practitioners, and laboratory technicians). Thus, physicians' use of
their titles in self-introductions may serve to clarify their identities as medical doctors. Moreover, as Richard Frankel notes (personal communication,
January 15, 1984), physicians in training may be particularly self-conscious
in their newly acquired roles. Hence, they may place more emphasis on
formal terms of address than do their older, more seasoned colleagues.

11. As indicated in the transcript of this fragment, the physician is looking at the patient as she delivers the news to which she summons his attention. He is not, for example, writing notes in her chart, or gazing out the
window. However, he offers neither a verbal nor non-verbal reaction to
her announcement, even in the two-second pause that follows it.

12. The addendum of "Miss" to a woman's first name might, of course,
be attributed to southern etiquette (e.g., "Miss Ellie," albeit a pseudonym
here, is also the usual form of address for a central character in the television series, *Dallas*). However, the physician involved in this particular exchange is not from the South, and his use of this addendum was occasional
rather than customary.

13. Differences in extent of acquaintanceship do not help account for
this finding. In all three cases, the patients were previously acquainted
with the physician and had sustained relationships with him for more than
a year.

14. A somewhat contrary finding is reported by Emerson (1970), who
observes that humor plays an important part in sustaining medical definitions of reality in gynecological examinations: "Humor may be used to
discount the line the patient is taking. At the same time, humor provides a
safety valve for all parties whereby the sexual connotations and general
concern about gynecological examinations may be expressed by indirec-
tion. . . . If a person can joke on a topic, he demonstrates to others that he
possesses a laudatory degree of detachment" (p. 89). However, since Emerson's analysis focuses on humor rather than laughter, and since she does
not provide quantitative details of her findings, it is difficult to compare
them with results reported here. It is possible that laughter occurs more

often in patients' encounters with gynecologists than in those with family physicians, but differences in Emerson's and my methods of analysis would make such a conclusion premature.

15. Coser's (1960) own results contradict the dominant perspective on humor. Her study of mental hospital staff meetings found that witticisms were distributed along the lines of the staff status hierarchy (with senior staff members initiating more humorous episodes than their junior colleagues). It is worth noting, however, that Coser's operational definition identifies a "witticism" as something that *elicits* laughter (p. 82). Thus, unsuccessful attempts at humor were not included in her analysis.

16. As Gilly West has pointed out to me, the avoidance of names by physician and patient also maintains an impersonal, clinical distance between parties involved, reducing interactions to exchanges between dispassionate clinicians and their clinical objects.

Chapter 8 Conclusions

1. Notable exceptions to this characterization are the earlier cited works dealing with the ongoing social construction of meanings in medical settings (e.g., Emerson, 1970; Ball, 1967; Becker et al., 1961; Freidson, 1961).

2. An important counter trend is suggested by the growing body of works that utilize discourse analytic techniques to pursue this topic (e.g., Cicourel, 1981a; 1981b; 1982; 1983; Fisher, 1983; Fisher and Todd, 1983a; 1983b; Labov and Fanshel, 1977; Måseide, 1983; Mishler, 1984; Paget, 1983; Tannen and Wallat, 1983; Todd, 1983).

3. To be sure, conversation analysis does have its critics (e.g., Cicourel, 1977; 1980b; Gumperz, 1982:158–160; Labov and Fanshel, 1977:24–27; Phillips, 1977). As should be clear from the earlier review of these works (see Chapter 2), discourse analyses stress the encoding and decoding of meaning in talk for individual speakers. Thus their interest in "technical" sequential account[s]" of talk's organization is a subsidiary interest—subordinated to concerns for "what is really going on interactionally" (Schegloff, 1980: 149–150). While I have severe reservations about many of the criticisms of conversation analysis here cited, this is not the place to address them in detail. Suffice it to say that I have employed this approach here in an effort to contribute to our understanding of talk between doctors and patients as a topic in its own right.

4. By "decision," I do not mean to imply a necessary *conscious* choice, but a process of selection from sets of alternative acts that constitute different states of talk.

5. The most fruitful applications of this perspective have actually analyzed physician-patient discourse as a resource for the construction of written medical records (see Cicourel, 1975; 1978; 1981a; 1983).

6. A word of caution is in order here. Some aspects of patients' health may only be established as "relevant" *after* conducting a review of symptoms (e.g., a review which yields a positive diagnosis). Even so, it is reasonable to ask: Is a review of symptoms always necessary? And, if it is necessary: Can it only be conducted through the chaining of questions and answers?

7. The title of this subsection is borrowed from Zimmerman and Pollner (1970).

8. My description is intended for physicians in the United States. However, evidence suggests that the socioeconomic status and prestige of physicians in this country are enjoyed by doctors throughout many Western societies (see Friedson, 1970b:173; Mechanic, 1979:177).

References

American Druggist
    1983   "Verbatim comments by RPh's about doctors who scribble." *American Druggist* (May): 64–68.

American Medical Association
    1973   *The Profile of Medical Practice*. Chicago: AMA Center for Health Services Research and Development.

Anderson, W. Timothy, and David T. Helm
    1979   "The physician-patient encounter: A process of reality negotiation." Pp. 259–271, in E. G. Jaco (ed.), *Patients, Physicians and Illness*. 3rd edition. New York: The Free Press.

Argyle, Michael, Mansur Lalljee, and Mark Cook
    1968   "The effects of visibility on interaction in a dyad." *Human Relations* 21:3–17.

Arms, Suzanne
    1975   *Immaculate Deception: A New Look at Women and Childbirth in America*. San Francisco and Boston: San Francisco Book Company/Houghton Mifflin.

Austin, John Langshaw
    1962   *How to Do Things with Words*. Cambridge: Harvard University Press.

Bain, D.J.G.
    1979   "The relationship between time and clinical management in Family Practice." *Journal of Family Practice* 8:551–559.

Bales, Robert F.
    1950   *Interaction Process Analysis: A Method for the Study of Small Groups*. Reading, Massachusetts: Addison-Wesley.

Ball, Donald W.
    1967   "An abortion clinic ethnography." *Social Problems* 14:293–301.

Banks, Franklin R., and Martin D. Keller
    1971   "Symptom experience and health action." *Medical Care* 9:498–502.

Becker, Howard S., Blanche Geer, Everett C. Hughes, and Anselm L. Strauss
    1961   *Boys in White: Student Culture in Medical School*. Chicago: University of Chicago Press.

Becker, Marshall H.
    1979   "Psychosocial aspects of health-related behavior." Pp. 253–274, in Howard E. Freeman, Sol Levine, and Leo G. Reeder (eds.), *Handbook of Medical Sociology*. 3rd edition. Englewood Cliffs, New Jersey: Prentice-Hall.

Belsky, Marvin S., and Leonard Gross
 1978 "Are you a smart patient?" *Cosmopolitan* 185:172 + .

Berger, Peter L., and Thomas Luckman
 1966 *The Social Construction of Reality: A Treatise in the Sociology of Knowledge.* Garden City, New York: Anchor/Doubleday.

Berkowitz, Norman H., Mary F. Malone, Malcolm W. Klein, and Ann Eaton
 1963 "Patient follow-through in the outpatient department." *Nursing Research* 12:16–22.

Berlin, Leonard
 1977 "How expert witnesses are shafting us." *Medical Economics* (November 14):121–128.

Bernard, Jessie
 1972 *The Sex Game.* New York: Atheneum.

Bloom, Samuel W.
 1963 *The Doctor and His Patient: A Sociological Interpretation.* New York: The Free Press.

Bloom, Samuel W., and Robert N. Wilson
 1979 "Patient-practitioner relationships." Pp. 275–296, in Howard E. Freeman, Sol Levine, and Leo G. Reeder (eds.), *Handbook of Medical Sociology.* 3rd edition. Englewood Cliffs, New Jersey: Prentice Hall.

Blumer, Herbert
 1969 *Symbolic Interactionism: Perspective and Method.* Englewood Cliffs, New Jersey: Prentice-Hall.

Bock, William, and Ross Egger
 1971 "The development of a behavioral science model for Family Practice." *Journal of Medical Education* 46:831–836.

Bookman, Ralph
 1984 Letter to the Editor. *American Medical News* (January 6):5.

Bosmajian, Haig
 1974 *The Language of Oppression.* Washington, D.C.: Public Affairs Press.

Boyle, Charles Murray
 1970 "Difference between patients' and doctors' interpretation of some common medical terms." *British Medical Journal* 2:286–289.

Braslow, Judith B., and Marilyn Heins
 1981 "Women in medical education: A decade of change." *New England Journal of Medicine* 304:1129–1135.

Brody, Barbara L., and Joseph Stokes III
 1970 "Use of professional time by Internists and General Practitioners in group and solo practice." *Annals of Internal Medicine* 73:741–749.

Brown, Roger
 1965 *Social Psychology.* New York: The Free Press.

Brown, Roger, and Marguerite Ford
 1961 "Address in American English." *Journal of Abnormal and Social Psychology* 62:375–385.

Brown, Roger, and Albert Gilman
1960   "The pronouns of power and solidarity." Pp. 253–276, in Thomas A. Sebeok (ed.), *Style in Language*. Jointly published by Technology Press of Massachusetts Institute of Technology and John Wiley and Sons, London.

Browne, Kevin, and Paul Freeling
1976   *The Doctor-Patient Relationship.* 2nd edition. London and Edinburgh: Churchill Livingstone.

Bucher, Rue, and Joan Stelling
1969   "Characteristics of professional organizations." *Journal of Health and Social Behavior* 10:3–15.

Byrne, Patrick S., and Barrie E. L. Long
1976   *Doctors Talking to Patients: A Study of the Verbal Behavior of General Practitioners Consulting in their Surgeries.* Southampton, England: Hobbs.

Cartwright, A., S. Lucas, and M. O'Brien
1974   *Exploring Communications in General Practice: A Feasibility Study.* Report to the Social Science Research Council, Institute for Social Studies in Medicine, London.

Chriss, Nicholas C.
1977   "Doctors down the logorrhea: De Bakey sisters cure 'medicalese.'" *Los Angeles Times* Part 1A p. 1–4, July 17, 1977.

Cicourel, Aaron V.
1975   "Discourse and text: Cognitive and linguistic processes in studies of social structure." *Versus: Quaderni di Studi Semotici* 12:33–84.

Cicourel, Aaron V.
1977   "Discourse, autonomous grammars and contextualized processing of information." Pp. 109–158, in *Proceedings of the Conference on the Analysis of Discourse.* Institut für Kommunikationsforschung und Phonetik, University of Bonn, Germany, October 14–16, 1976. Hamburg: Helmut Buske Verlag.

Cicourel, Aaron V.
1978   "Language and society: Cognitive, cultural and linguistic aspects of language use." *Sozialwissenschaftliche Annalen,* Band 2, Seite B25-B58. Physica-Verlag: Vienna.

Cicourel, Aaron V.
1980a   "Language and social interaction: Philosophical and empirical issues." *Sociological Inquiry* 50:1–30.

Cicourel, Aaron V.
1980b   "Three models of discourse analysis: The role of social structure." *Discourse Processes* 3:101–132.

Cicourel, Aaron V.
1981a   "Language and medicine." Pp. 407–429, in C. Ferguson and S. Brice Heath (eds.), *Language in the USA.* Cambridge: Cambridge University Press.

Cicourel, Aaron V.
1981b   "The role of cognitive-linguistic concepts in understanding everyday social interactions." *Annual Review of Sociology* 7:87–106.

Cicourel, Aaron V.
1982   "Language and belief in a medical setting." Pp. 48–78, in H.
            Byrnes (ed.), Georgetown University Roundtable on Lan-
            guages and Linguistics (1982). *Contemporary Perceptions of
            Language: Interdisciplinary Dimensions.* Georgetown, Washing-
            ton: Georgetown University Press.
Cicourel, Aaron V.
1983   "Hearing is not believing: Language and the structure of
            belief in medical communication." Pp. 221–239, in S. Fisher
            and A. D. Todd (eds.), *The Social Organization of Doctor-Patient
            Communication.* Washington, D.C.: Center for Applied
            Linguistics.
Collins, G. E.
1955   "Do we really advise the patient?" *Journal of the Florida Medi-
            cal Association* 42:111–115.
Conant, Elizabeth Babbott
1983   "Addressing patients by their names." *New England Journal of
            Medicine* 308 (January 27):226.
Conrad, Peter, and Rochelle Kern (eds.)
1981   *The Sociology of Health and Illness.* New York: St. Martin's
            Press.
Corea, Gena
1978   *The Hidden Malpractice: How American Medicine Mistreats
            Women.* New York: Jove/Harcourt Brace Jovanovich.
Coser, Rose Laub
1959   "Some social functions of laughter." *Human Relations* 12:171–
            182.
Coser, Rose Laub
1960   "Laughter among colleagues: A study of the social functions
            of humor among the staff of a mental hospital." *Psychiatry*
            23:81–95.
Croog, Sydney H.
1961   "Ethnic origins, educational level, and responses to a health
            questionnaire." *Human Organization* 20:65–69.
Curry, Hiram B.
1979   "Decline of General Practice; Birth of Family Practice." Un-
            published manuscript. Department of Family Practice, Med-
            ical University of South Carolina, Charleston.
Daly, Mary
1978   *Gyn/Ecology: The Metaethics of Radical Feminism.* Boston: Bea-
            con Press.
Daniels, Arlene Kaplan
1973   "The philosophy of combat psychiatry." Pp. 132–140, in E.
            Rubington and M. S. Weinburg (eds.), *Deviance: The Interac-
            tionist Perspective.* New York: Macmillan.
Danziger, Sandra Klein
1980   "The medical model in doctor-patient interaction: The case
            of pregnancy care." Pp. 263–304, in J. Roth (ed.), *Research in
            the Sociology of Health Care.* Greenwich, Connecticut: JAI
            Press.

Danziger, Sandra Klein

1981 "The uses of expertise in doctor-patient encounters during pregnancy." Pp. 359–376, in P. Conrad and R. Kern (eds.), *The Sociology of Health and Illness: Critical Perspectives*. New York: St. Martin's Press. (Originally published in *Social Science and Medicine* 12:359–367, 1978.)

Davis, Fred

1964 "Deviance disavowal: The management of strained interaction by the visibly physically handicapped." Pp. 119–137 in H. Becker (ed.), *The Other Side*. New York: The Free Press.

Davis, J. Mostyn

1978 "Little ways to save a lot of time." *Medical Economics* (March 20):93–113.

Davis, Milton S.

1968 "Variations in patients' compliance with doctors' advice: An empirical analysis of patterns of communication." *American Journal of Public Health* 58:274–288.

Delamont, Sara, and David Hamilton

1976 "Classroom research: A critique and a new approach." Pp. 3–, in M. Stubbs and S. Delamont (eds.), *Explorations in Classroom Observation*. London: John Wiley and Sons.

Derbyshire, Robert C.

1977 "Review of *The Unkindest Cut*, by Marcia Millman." *Hospital Practice* (April):133.

Dreifus, Claudia (ed.)

1977 *Seizing Our Bodies: The Politics of Women's Health*. New York: Vintage Books.

Eakins, Barbara Westbrook, and R. Gene Eakins

1976 *Sex Differences in Human Communication*. Boston: Houghton Mifflin.

Ehrenreich, Barbara, and Deirdre English

1978 *For Her Own Good: 150 Years of the Experts' Advice to Women*. Garden City, New York: Anchor Press/Doubleday.

Ekman, Paul

1980 *Face of Man: Universal Expression in a New Guinea Village*. New York: Garland.

Ekman, Paul, and Wallace V. Frieson

1969 "The repertoire of nonverbal behavior: Categories, origins, usage and coding." *Semiotica* 1:63–68.

Elling, Ray, Ruth Whittemore, and Morris Green

1960 "Patient participation in a Pediatric program." *Journal of Health and Human Behavior* 1:183–191.

Emerson, Joan P.

1970 "Behavior in private places: Sustaining definitions of reality in gynecological examinations." Pp. 74–97, in H. P. Dreitzel (ed.), *Recent Sociology No. 2*. New York: Macmillan.

Fee, Elizabeth (ed.)

1975 *Women and Health: The Politics of Sex in Medicine*. Farmingdale, New York: Baywood Publishing.

Feldman, Jacob J.
    1966   *The Dissemination of Health Information: A Case Study in Adult Learning.* Chicago: Aldine.
Fischl, Robert A.
    1976   "Take credit for what you do for the patient." *Medical Economics* (November 15):231–236.
Fisher, John J.
    1977   "Who's in charge here, anyway?" *Medical Economics* (May 16):169.
Fisher, Sue
    1983   "Doctor talk/patient talk: How treatment decisions are negotiated in doctor-patient communication." Pp. 135–157, in S. Fisher and A. D. Todd (eds.), *The Social Organization of Doctor-Patient Communication.* Washington, D.C.: Center for Applied Linguistics.
Fisher, Sue, and Alexandra Dundas Todd
    1983a   "Friendly persuasion: The negotiation of decisions to use oral contraceptives." Paper presented at the American Sociological Association Annual Meeting, Detroit, Michigan (August).
Fisher, Sue, and Alexandra Dundas Todd
    1983b   "Introduction: Communication and social context—toward broader definitions." Pp. 3–17, in S. Fisher and A. D. Todd (eds.), *The Social Organization of Doctor-Patient Communication.*" Washington, D.C.: Center for Applied Linguistics.
Flanders, Ned A.
    1970   *Analyzing Teaching Behavior.* Reading, Massachusetts: Addison-Wesley.
Francis, Vida, Barbara M. Korsch, and Marie J. Morris
    1969   "Gaps in doctor-patient communication: Patients' response to medical advice." *New England Journal of Medicine* 280:535–540.
Frankel, Richard M.
    1982   "Autism for all practical purposes: A micro-interactional view." *Topics in Language Disorders* 3:33–42.
Frankel, Richard M.
    1983   "The laying on of hands: Aspects of the organization of gaze, touch, and talk in a medical encounter." Pp. 19–54, in S. Fisher and A. D. Todd (eds.), *The Social Organization of Doctor-Patient Communication.* Washington, D.C.: Center for Applied Linguistics.
Frankel, Richard M.
    1984   "From sentence to 'sequence': Understanding the medical encounter through microinteractional analysis." *Discourse Processes* 7:135–170.
Frankel, Richard M.
    (in   "Talking in interviews: A dispreference for patient-initiated
    press)   questions in physician-patient encounters." In G. Psathas (ed.), *Interactional Competence.* New York: Irvington.

Frankel, Richard M.
(forth-   "Microanalysis and the medical encounter: An exploratory
coming)   study." In D. Helm, W. T. Anderson, and A. J. Meehan (eds.),
             New Directions in Ethnomethodology and Conversation Analysis.
             New York: Irvington.
Frankel, Richard M.
(in prep-   *Telling Concerns: Social Interaction in Medical Encounters.* Mon-
aration)   ograph to appear in the C. Wallet and J. Green (eds.) series,
             Language and Learning in the Human Service Professions. Nor-
             wood, New Jersey: Ablex.
Frankel, Richard M., and Howard B. Beckman
1981   "Closing up openings: An analysis of the presenting com-
             plaint in medical encounters." Paper presented at the 6th
             Annual International Institute in Ethnomethodology and
             Conversation Analysis, Boston (August).
Frankel, Richard M., and Howard B. Beckman
1982   "Impact: An interaction-based method for preserving and
             analyzing clinical transactions." Pp. 71–85, in L. S. Pettigrew
             (ed.), *Explorations in Provider and Patient Interaction.* Louis-
             ville, Kentucky: Humana, Inc.
Frazer, James
1951   *The Golden Bough.* New York: Macmillan.
Freemon, Barbara, Vida F. Negrete, Milton Davis, and Barbara M. Korsch
1971   "Gaps in doctor-patient communication: Doctor-patient in-
             teraction analysis." *Pediatric Research* 5:298–311.
Freidson, Eliot
1961   *Patients' Views of Medical Practice—A Study of Subscribers to a
             Prepaid Medical Plan in the Bronx.* New York: Russell Sage
             Foundation.
Freidson, Eliot
1970a   *Professional Dominance: The Social Structure of Medical Care.*
             New York: Atherton Press.
Freidson, Eliot
1970b   *Profession of Medicine: A Study of the Sociology of Applied Knowl-
             edge.* New York: Harper & Row.
Freidson, Eliot
1975   *Doctoring Together: A Study of Professional Social Control.* New
             York: Elsevier.
Funk and Wagnalls
1964   *Funk and Wagnalls Standard Dictionary.* Britannica World Lan-
             guage edition. Volume 2. New York: Funk and Wagnalls.
Galton, Lawrence
1979   "Often-missed diagnoses: A guide to mystery ailments." *Fam-
             ily Circle* 92 (March):8 + .
Glaser, Barney G., and Anselm Strauss
1965   "Temporal aspects of dying as a nonscheduled status pas-
             sage." *American Journal of Sociology* 71:45–69.
Goffman, Erving
1967   *Interaction Ritual: Essays on Face-to-Face Behavior.* Garden City,
             New York: Anchor Books.

Goffman, Erving
 1979   *Gender Advertisements.* New York: Harper Colophon Books.
             (Originally published in *Studies in the Anthropology of Visual
             Communication* 3, no. 2, 1976.)
Goffman, Erving
 1981a   "Radio talk." Pp. 197–330, in E. Goffman, *Forms of Talk.* Phil-
             adelphia: University of Pennsylvania Press.
Goffman, Erving
 1981b   "Replies and responses." Pp. 5–77, in E. Goffman, *Forms of
             Talk.* Philadelphia: University of Pennsylvania Press. (Origi-
             nally published in *Language in Society* 5:257–313, 1976.)
Goodwin, Charles
 1980   "Restarts, pauses and the achievement of a state of mutual
             gaze at turn-beginning." *Sociological Inquiry* 50:277–302.
Goodwin, Charles
 1981   *Conversational Organization: Interaction between speakers and
             hearers.* New York: Academic Press.
Goodwin, Marjorie Harness
 1980   "Processes of mutual monitoring implicated in the produc-
             tion of description sequences." *Sociological Inquiry* 50:303–
             317.
Gordon, Linda
 1976   *Woman's Body, Woman's Right: A Social History of Birth Control
             in America.* Middlesex, England: Penguin Books.
Gottschalk, Louis A., and Goldine C. Gleser
 1969   *The Measurement of Psychological States Through the Content
             Analysis of Verbal Behavior.* Berkeley: University of California
             Press.
Grimshaw, Allen
 1980   "Mishearings, misunderstandings and other nonsuccesses in
             talk: A plea for redress of a speaker-oriented bias." *Sociologi-
             cal Inquiry* 50:31–74.
Gumperz, John J.
 1972   "Sociolinguistics and communication in small groups." Pp.
             203–224, in J. B. Pride and J. Holmes (eds.), *Sociolinguistics.*
             Baltimore: Penguin.
Gumperz, John J.
 1982   *Discourse Strategies.* New York, Cambridge University Press.
Guttmacher, Sally, and Jack Elinson
 1971   "Ethno-religious variation in perceptions of illness." *Social
             Science and Medicine* 5:117–125.
Hayes-Bautista, David E.
 1978   "Chicano patients and medical practitioners: A sociology of
             knowledges paradigm of lay-professional interaction." *Social
             Science and Medicine* 12:83–90.
Heath, Christian C.
 1981   "The opening sequence in doctor-patient interaction." Pp.
             71–89, in C. C. Heath and P. Atkinson (eds.), *Medical Work:
             Realities and Routines.* Aldershot, England: Gower.

Heath, Christian C.
1982a   "Preserving the consultation: Medical cards and professional conduct." *The Journal of the Sociology of Health and Illness* 4:56–74.

Heath, Christian C.
1982b   "The maintenance of participation in social interaction." Paper presented at the International Sociological Association Xth World Congress in Sociology. Mexico City (August).

Heath, Christian C.
(in press)   "The display of recipiency: An instance of a sequential relationship in speech and body movement." To appear in *Semiotica.*

Heath, Christian C.
(forth-coming)   "Gaze solicitation and next speaker selection." To appear in the *International Journal of the Sociology of Language.*

Henley, Nancy M.
1977   *Body Politics: Power, Sex and Nonverbal Communication.* Englewood Cliffs, New Jersey: Prentice Hall.

Hetherington, Robert W., and Carl E. Hopkins
1969   "Symptom sensitivity: Its social and cultural correlates." *Health Services Research* 4:63–70.

Hogan, Patricia
1978   "A woman is not a girl and other lessons in corporate speech." Pp. 168–172, in B. A. Stead (ed.), *Women in Management.* Englewood Cliffs, New Jersey: Prentice-Hall.

Horsley, Jack E., with John H. Lavin
1977   "An up-to-date guide to informed consent." *Medical Economics* (March 21):150–169.

Hughes, Everett C.
1945   "Dilemmas and contradictions of status." *American Journal of Sociology* 50:353–354.

Hughes, Everett C.
1958   *Men and Their Work.* New York: The Free Press.

Hughes, Everett C.
1971   *The Sociological Eye: Selected Papers on Work, Self and the Study of Society.* Chicago: Aldine.

Hymes, Dell
1974   *Foundations in Sociolinguistics: An Ethnographic Approach.* Philadelphia: University of Pennsylvania Press.

Hymes, Dell (ed.)
1964   *Language in Culture and Society.* New York: Harper & Row.

Jefferson, Gail
1971   "A report on some difficulties encountered when using pseudonyms in research generative transcripts." Unpublished manuscript, Department of Social Relations, University of California, Irvine.

Jefferson, Gail
1972   "Side sequences." Pp. 294–338, in D. Sudnow (ed.), *Studies in Social Interaction.* New York: The Free Press.

Jefferson, Gail
    1973   "A case of precision timing in ordinary conversation: Over-
                lapped tag-positioned address terms in closing sequences."
                Semiotica IX: 47–96.
Jefferson, Gail
    1979   "A technique for inviting laughter and its subsequent accept-
                ance/declination." Pp. 23–78, in G. Psathas (ed.), *Everyday
                Language: Studies in Ethnomethodology.* New York: Irvington.
Jefferson, Gail and Emanuel A. Schegloff
    1975   "Sketch: Some orderly aspects of overlap in natural conver-
                sation." Unpublished manuscript, Department of Sociology,
                University of California, Los Angeles.
Kendon, Adam
    1981   *Nonverbal Communication, Interaction, and Gesture.* The Hague:
                Mouton.
Korsch, Barbara M., Ethel K. Gozzi, and Vida Francis Negrete
    1968   "Gaps in doctor-patient interaction and patient satisfaction."
                Pediatrics 42:855–870.
Korsch, Barbara M., and Vida Francis Negrete
    1972   "Doctor-patient communication." *Scientific American* 227:66–
                74.
Kramarae, Cheris
    1981   *Women and Men Speaking.* Rowley, Massachusetts: Newbury
                House.
Kramer, Cheris
    1975   "Women's speech: Separate but unequal?" Pp. 43–56, in B.
                Thorne and N. Henley (eds.), *Language and Sex: Difference
                and Dominance.* Rowley, Massachusetts: Newbury House.
Labov, William, and David Fanshel
    1977   *Therapeutic Discourse: Psychotherapy as Conversation.* New York:
                Academic Press.
Lakoff, Robin
    1975   *Language and Woman's Place.* New York: Harper Colophon.
Lavin, John H.
    1977   "Stay healthy—or else." *Medical Economics* (December 12):
                171–178.
Laws, Judith Long
    1971   "A feminist review of marital adjustment literature: The rape
                of the Locke." *Journal of Marriage and the Family* 33:483–516.
Lennard, Henry L., and Arnold Bernstein
    1960   *The Anatomy of Psychotherapy.* New York: Columbia University
                Press.
Leventhal, Howard
    1965   "Fear communications in the acceptance of preventative
                health practices." *Bulletin of the New York Academy of Medicine*
                41:1144–1168.
Lewy, Robert M.
    1977   "The emergence of the family practitioner: An historical
                analysis of a new speciality." *Journal of Medical Education*
                52:873–881.

Ley, Philip
1983 "Patients' understanding and recall in clinical communication failure." Pp. 89–107, in D. Pendleton and J. Nasler (eds.), *Doctor-Patient Communication*. London: Academic Press.

Ley, P., and M. S. Spelman
1965 "Communications in an outpatient setting." *British Journal of Social and Clinical Psychology* 4:114–116.

Ley, P., and M. S. Spelman
1967 *Communicating with the Patient*. St. Louis: Warren H. Green.

Lorber, Judith
1975 "Women and medical sociology: Invisible professionals and ubiquitous patients." Pp. 75–105, in M. Millman and R. M. Kanter (eds.), *Another Voice: Feminist Perspectives on Social Life and Social Science*. Garden City, New York: Anchor Press/ Doubleday.

Luker, Kristin
1976 *Taking Chances: Abortion and the Decision Not to Contracept*. Berkeley: University of California Press.

Luker, Kristin
1984 *Abortion and the Politics of Motherhood*. Berkeley: University of California Press.

Lukomnik, Joanne
1978 "Family practice: Teaching old docs new tricks?" *Health/PAC Bulletin* 80:2–31.

Måseide, Per
1983 "Analytical aspects of clinical reasoning: A discussion of models for medical problem solving." Pp. 241–265, in S. Fisher and A. D. Todd (eds.), *The Social Organization of Doctor-Patient Communication*. Washington, D.C.: Center for Applied Linguistics.

Mattera, Marianne Dekker
1980 "Female doctors: Why they're on an economic treadmill." *Medical Economics* (February 18):98–110.

McCauley, Mary H.
1978 "Application of the Myers-Briggs type indicator to medicine and other health professions." Unpublished manuscript. The Center for Applications of Psychological Type, Gainesville, Florida.

McKinlay, John B.
1975 "Who is really ignorant?—physician or patient." *Journal of Health and Social Behavior* 16:3–11.

McMillan, Leslie R., A. Kay Clifton, Diane McGrath, and Wanda S. Gale
1977 "Women's language: Uncertainty or interpersonal sensitivity and emotionality?" *Sex Roles* 3:545–559.

Mechanic, David
1972 "Social psychological factors affecting the presentation of bodily complaints." *New England Journal of Medicine* 286:1132–1139.

Mechanic, David
  1979   "Physicians." Pp. 177–192, in H. E. Freeman, S. Levine, and
            L. G. Reeder (eds.), *Handbook of Medical Sociology.* 3rd edition.
            Englewood Cliffs, New Jersey: Prentice-Hall.
Meehan, Albert J.
  1981   "Some conversational features of the use of medical terms by
            doctors and patients in interaction." Pp. 107–127, in P. Atkin-
            son and C. C. Heath (eds.), *Medical Work: Realities and Rou-
            tines.* Farnborough, England: Gower.
Mehr, Michael
  1984   Letter to the Editor. *American Medical News* (January 6):5.
Miller, Casey, and Kate Swift
  1977   *Words and Women.* Garden City, New York: Anchor Books.
Millman, Marcia
  1977   *The Unkindest Cut: Life in the Backrooms of Medicine.* New York:
            William Morrow & Co.
Mishler, Elliott G.
  1979   "Meaning in context: Is there any other kind?" *Harvard Edu-
            cational Review* 49:1–19.
Mishler, Elliott G.
  1984   *The Discourse of Medicine: Dialectics of Medical Interviews.* Nor-
            wood, New Jersey: Ablex Publishing.
Natale, Michael, Elliot Entin, and Joseph Jaffee
  1979   "Vocal interruptions in dyadic communication as a function
            of speech and social anxiety." *Journal of Personality and Social
            Psychology* 37:865–878.
National NOW Times
  1983   "In Brief." *National NOW Times* (May):2.
Natkins, Lucille G.
  1983   "Hi, Lucille, this is Dr. Gold!" *Ms.* (February):104. (Originally
            published in the *Journal of the American Medical Association* 247
            [May 7, 1982].)
Neumann, Hans H.
  1977   "The next big malpractice risk." *Medical Economics* (Novem-
            ber 28):80–86.
Nierenberg, Judith, and Florence Janovic
  1979   "Guide to Medical Language." *Family Circle* 92(1):49–50.
            (Excerpted from J. Nierenberg and F. Janovic, *The Hospital
            Experience.* Indianapolis, Indiana: Bobbs-Merrill, 1978.)
Octigan, Mary, and Sharon Niederman
  1979   "Male dominance in conversation." *Frontiers* 4:50–54.
Paget, Marianne A.
  1983   "On the work of talk: Studies in misunderstandings." Pp. 55–
            74, in S. Fisher and A. D. Todd (eds.), *The Social Organization
            of Doctor-Patient Communication.* Washington, D.C.: Center for
            Applied Linguistics.
Pantell, Robert H., Thomas J. Stewart, James K. Dias, Patricia Wells, and
A. William Ross
  1982   "Physician communication with children and parents." *Pedi-
            atrics* 70:396–402.

Parchini, Allan
1983 "Doctors: Familiarity breeds contempt." *Los Angeles Times* (February 1): Part V, 1–2.
Parrish, Henry M., F. Marian Bishop, and A. Sherwood Baker
1967 "Time study of general practioners' office hours." *Archives of Environmental Health* 14:892–898.
Parsons, Talcott
1951 *The Social System.* New York: The Free Press.
Parsons, Talcott
1975 "The sick role and the role of the physician reconsidered." *Millbank Memorial Fund Quarterly* 53:257–277.
Parsons, Talcott, and Renee Fox
1952 "Illness, therapy and the modern urban American family." *Journal of Social Issues* 8:31–44.
Pendleton, David
1983 "Doctor-patient communication: A review." Pp. 5–53, in D. Pendleton and John Hasler (eds.), *Doctor-Patient Communication.* London: Academic Press.
Pendleton, David A., and Stephen Bochner
1980 "The communication of medical information in general practice consultations as a function of patients' social class." *Social Science and Medicine* 14A:669–673.
Phillips, Susan Urmston
1977 "Some sources of cultural variability in the regulation of talk." *Language in Society* 5:81–95.
Rakel, Robert E.
1977 *Principles of Family Medicine.* Philadelphia: W. B. Saunders Co.
Random House, Inc.
1975 *Random House College Dictionary.* Revised edition. New York: Random House.
Ray, Michael L., and Eugene J. Webb
1966 "Speech duration effects in the Kennedy news conferences." *Science* 153:899–901.
Redlich, Frederick C.
1945 "The patient's language: An investigation into the use of medical terms." *Yale Journal of Biology and Medicine* 17:427–453.
Reeder, Leo G.
1972 "The patient-client as a consumer: Some observations on the changing professional-client relationship." *Journal of Health and Social Behavior* 13:406–412.
Robertson, Dwight L.
1981 "Symptoms offered during a three year family practice residency experience." *Journal of Family Practice* 13:239–244.
Robillard, Albert B., Geoffrey M. White, and Thomas W. Maretzki
1983 "Between doctor and patient: Informed consent in conversational interaction." Pp. 107–134, in S. Fisher and A. D. Todd (eds.), *The Social Organization of Doctor-Patient Communication.* Washington, D.C.: Center for Applied Linguistics.

Rosenberg, Charlotte L.
1977   "Nine experts pinpoint the most common practice errors."
           Medical Economics (November 14):98–108.
Roter, Deborah L.
1977   "Patient participation in the patient-provider interaction:
           The effects of patient question-asking on the quality of inter-
           action, satisfaction and compliance." *Health Education Mono-
           graphs* 5:281–315.
Roth, Julius
1963a   "Information and the control of treatment in tuberculosis
           hospitals." Pp. 293–317, in E. Freidson (ed.), *The Hospital in
           Modern Society.* New York: The Free Press.
Roth, Julius
1963b   *Timetables.* Indianapolis: Bobbs Merrill.
Rowen, Manuel J.
1977   "Do you always hear out your patients? I don't." *Medical Eco-
           nomics* (December 26):82–86.
Royal College of General Practitioners
1972   *The Future General Practitioner: Teaching and Learning.* Lon-
           don: Royal College of General Practitioners.
Ruzek, Sheryl Burt
1979   *The Women's Health Movement.* New York: Praeger.
Sacks, Harvey
1963   "On sociological description." *Berkeley Journal of Sociology*
           8:1–16.
Sacks, Harvey
1966   Unpublished lectures. Department of Sociology, University
           of California, Los Angeles.
Sacks, Harvey
1972   "On the analyzability of stories by children." Pp. 325–345, in
           J. J. Gumperz and D. Hymes (eds.), *Directions in Sociolinguis-
           tics: The Ethnography of Communication.* New York: Holt, Rine-
           hart and Winston.
Sacks, Harvey, Emanuel A. Schegloff, and Gail Jefferson
1974   "A simplest systematics for the organization of turn-taking
           for conversation." *Language* 50:696–735.
Saroyn, William
1953   "Random notes on the names of people." *Names* 1:239–241.
Scheff, Thomas J.
1963   "Negotiating reality: Notes on power in the assessment of
           responsibility." *Social Problems* 16:3–17.
Scheflin, Albert E.
1972   *Body Language and Social Order.* Englewood Cliffs, New Jer-
           sey: Prentice-Hall.
Schegloff, Emanuel A.
1968   "Sequencing in conversational openings." *American Anthropol-
           ogist* 70:1075–1095.
Schegloff, Emanuel A.
1972   "Notes on a conversational practice: Formulating place." Pp.
           75–119, in D. Sundow (ed.), *Studies in Social Interaction.* New
           York: The Free Press.

Schegloff, Emanuel A.
1979   "The relevance of repair to syntax-for-conversation." *Syntax and Semantics* 12: *Discourse and Syntax* 261–286.
Schegloff, Emanuel A.
1980   "Preliminaries to preliminaries: "Can I ask you a question?" *Sociological Inquiry* 50:104–152.
Schegloff, Emanuel A.
1981   "Discourse as an interactional achievement." Paper presented at the Georgetown University Roundtable on Linguistics and Language Studies. March, 1981.
Schegloff, Emanuel A., Gail Jefferson, and Harvey Sacks
1977   "The preference for self-correction in the organization of repair in conversation." *Language* 53:361–382.
Schegloff, Emanuel A., and Harvey Sacks
1974   "Opening up closings." Pp. 233–264, in R. Turner (ed.), *Ethnomethodology: Selected Readings.* Baltimore: Penguin. (Originally published in *Semiotica* 8:289–327, 1973.)
Scherer, Klaus, and Paul Ekman (eds.)
1982   *Handbook of Methods in Nonverbal Behavior Research.* Cambridge: Cambridge University Press.
Schwarz, Barry
1974   "Waiting, exchange and power: The distribution of time in social systems." *American Journal of Sociology* 79:841–870.
Scully, Diana
1980   *Men Who Control Women's Health: The Miseducation of Obstetrician-Gynecologists.* Boston: Houghton Mifflin.
Seaman, Barbara
1969   *The Doctors' Case Against the Pill.* New York: Avon.
Seaman, Barbara, and Gideon Seaman
1977   *Women and the Crisis in Sex Hormones.* New York: Bantam.
Seligmann, Arthur W., Neva Eileen McGrath, and Lois Pratt
1957   "Level of medical information among clinic patients." *Journal of Chronic Diseases* 6:497–509.
Shapiro, Eileen C., Florence P. Haseltine, and Mary P. Rowe
1978   "Moving up: Role models, mentors, and the 'Patron System.'" *Sloan Management Review* 19:51–58.
Shaw, Nancy Stoller
1974   *Forced Labor: Maternity Care in the United States.* New York: Pergamon Press.
Shuy, Roger
1976   "The medical interview: Problems in communication." *Primary Care* 3:365–386.
Shuy, Roger
1983   "Three types of interference to an effective exchange of information in the medical interview." Pp. 189–202, in S. Fisher and A. D. Todd (eds.), *The Social Organization of Doctor-Patient Communication.* Washington, D.C.: Center for Applied Linguistics.
Siegel, Irwin M.
1977   "The patient with the little paper—and all the rest." *Medical Economics* (August 8):149–159.

Silver, Johnathan M.
1979   "Medical terms—A two-way block?" *Colloquy: The Journal of Physician-Patient Communications* (November)4–10.

Simon, Anita, and E. Gil Boyer
1968   *Mirrors for Behavior.* Philadelphia: Research for Better Schools.

Skipper, James K.
1965   "Communication and the hospitalized patient." Pp. 61–82, in J. K. Skipper and R. C. Leonard (eds.), *Social Interaction and Patient Care.* Philadelphia: Lippincott.

Slater, Phillip
1961   "Parental role differentiation." *American Journal of Sociology* 67:296–311.

Stewart, Moira A., Ian R. McWhinney, and Carol W. Buck
1975   "How illness presents: A study of patient behavior." *The Journal of Family Practice* 2:411–414.

Stewart, Thomas J., A. William Ross, James K. Dias, and Robert H. Pantell
1980   "Child, parent and physician communication in Family Practice." Unpublished manuscript. Department of Family Medicine, Medical University of South Carolina, Charleston.

Stoeckle, John D., Irving Kenneth Zola, and Gerald E. Davidson
1963   "On going to see the doctor: The contributions of the patient to the decision to seek medical aid: A selected review." *Journal of Chronic Diseases* 16:975–989.

Stoeckle, John D., Irving Kenneth Zola, and Gerald E. Davidson
1964   "The quantity and significance of psychological distress in medical patients—some preliminary observations about the decision to seek medical aid." *Journal of Chronic Diseases* 17:959–970.

Stone, George C.
1979   "Patient compliance and the role of the expert." *Journal of Social Issues* 35:34–59.

Strauss, Anselm L.
1970   *Where Medicine Fails.* Chicago: Aldine.

Stromberg, Ann (ed.)
1984   *Women, Health and Medicine.* Palo Alto: Mayfield.

Strong, P. M.
1979   *The Ceremonial Order of the Clinic: Parents, Doctors and Medical Bureaucracies.* London: Routledge & Kegan Paul.

Svarstad, Bonnie L.
1979   "Physician-patient communication and patient conformity with medical advice." Pp. 243–259, in G. L. Albrecht and P. C. Higgins (eds.), *Health, Illness and Medicine: A Reader in Medical Sociology.* Chicago: Rand McNally. (Originally pp. 220–238, in D. Mechanic (ed.), *The Growth of Bureaucratic Medicine.* New York: John Wiley & Sons, 1976.)

Svarstad, Bonnie L., and Helene Levens Lipton
1977   "Informing parents about mental retardation: A study of professional communication and parent acceptance." *Social Science and Medicine* 11:645–651.

Szasz, Thomas, and Marc Hollender
  1956 "A contribution to the philosophy of medicine: The basic models of the doctor-patient relationship." *Journal of the American Medical Association* 97:585–588.

Tannen, Deborah
  (in   "Frames and schemas in sociolinguistic analysis of pediatric
  press) interaction." *Quaderni di Semantica.*

Tannen, Deborah, and Cynthia Wallat
  1983 "Doctor/mother/child communication: Linguistic analysis of a pediatric interaction." Pp. 203–220, in S. Fisher and A. D. Todd (eds.), *The Social Organization of Doctor-Patient Communication.* Washington, D.C.: Center for Applied Linguistics.

Thomas, Sari
  1980 "Audience soundmaking." Paper presented at the 30th Annual Meeting of the American Anthropological Association, Washington, D.C.

Thorne, Barrie
  1980 " 'You still takin' notes?' Fieldwork and problems of informed consent." *Social Problems* 27:284–297.

Thorne, Barrie, and Nancy Henley (eds.)
  1975 *Language and Sex: Difference and Dominance.* Rowley, Massachusetts: Newbury House.

Todd, Alexandra Dundas
  1983 "A diagnosis of doctor-patient discourse in the prescription of contraception." Pp. 159–187, in S. Fisher and A. D. Todd (eds.), *The Social Organization of Doctor-Patient Communication.* Washington, D.C.: Center for Applied Linguistics.

Trudgill, Peter
  1974 *Sociolinguistics: An Introduction.* Middlesex, England: Penguin Books.

U.S. Department of Health, Education and Welfare
  1983a "1981 Summary: National Ambulatory Medical Care Survey." *Advance Data* 88 (March 16):1–10.

U.S. Department of Health, Education and Welfare
  1983b "Drug Utilization in General and Family Practice by Characteristics of Physicians and Office Visits: National Ambulatory Medical Care Survey, 1980." *Advance Data* 87 (March 28):1–12.

Veatch, Robert M.
  1977 Interviewed in "Coping with today's ethical dilemmas: Part 2." *Medical Economics* (December 12):82–104.

Waitzkin, Howard
  1979 "Medicine, superstructure and micropolitics." *Social Science and Medicine* 13A:601–609.

Waitzkin, Howard
  1983 *The Second Sickness: Contradictions of Capitalist Health Care.* New York: The Free Press.

Waitzkin, Howard, and John D. Stoeckle
  1976 "Information control and the micro-politics of health care: Summary of an ongoing research project." *Social Science and Medicine* 10:263–276.

Wallen, Jacqueline, Howard Waitzkin, and John D. Stoeckle
1979   "Physician stereotypes about female health and illness: A study of patients' sex and the informative process during medical interviews." *Women and Health* 4:135–146.

Walsh, Mary Roth
1977   *Doctors Wanted: No Women Need Apply.* New Haven: Yale University Press.

Wertz, Richard W., and Dorothy C. Wertz
1977   *Lying-In: A History of Childbirth in America.* New York: Schocken Books.

West, Candace
1978   "Communicating Gender: A Study of Dominance and Control in Conversation." Unpublished doctoral dissertation. Department of Sociology, University of California, Santa Barbara.

West, Candace
1979   "Against our will: Male interruptions of females in cross-sex conversation." *Annals of the New York Academy of Sciences* 327:81–97.

West, Candace
1982   "Why can't a woman be more like a man? An interactional note on organizational game-playing for managerial women." *Sociology of Work and Occupations* 9:5–29.

West, Candace
1983   " 'Ask me no questions . . .' An analysis of queries and replies in physician-patient dialogues." Pp. 75–106, in S. Fisher and A. D. Todd (eds.), *The Social Organization of Doctor-Patient Communication.* Washington, D.C.: Center for Applied Linguistics.

West, Candace
1984   "Medical misfires: Mishearings, misgivings and misunderstandings in physician-patient dialogues." *Discourse Processes* 7:107–134.

West, Candace, and Sofia Gruskin
1982   "Doctor-patient dialogues: No laughing matters." Presented to the Annual Conference of the International Communication Association, Boston, Massachusetts (May).

West, Candace, and Don H. Zimmerman
1977   "Women's place in everyday talk: Reflections on parent-child interaction." *Social Problems* 24:521–529.

West, Candace, and Don H. Zimmerman
1982   "Conversation analysis." Pp. 506–541, in K. R. Scherer and P. Ekman (eds.), *Handbook of Methods in Nonverbal Behavior Research.* New York: Cambridge University Press.

West, Candace, and Don H. Zimmerman
1983   "Small insults: A study of interruptions in cross-sex conversations between unacquainted persons." Pp. 86–111, in B. Thorne, C. Kramarae, and N. Henley (eds.), *Language, Gender and Society.* Rowley, Massachusetts: Newbury House.

Willis, Frank N., and Sharon J. Williams
1976   "Simultaneous talking in conversation and sex of speakers."
        Perceptual and Motor Skills 43:1067–70.
Wilson, Robert N.
1970   *The Sociology of Health: An Introduction.* New York: Random
        House.
Wolinsky, Frederic D.
1980   *The Sociology of Health: Principles, Professions and Issues.* Bos-
        ton: Little, Brown and Company.
Zborowski, Mark
1958   "Cultural components in responses to pain." *Journal of Social
        Issues* 8:16–30.
Zimmerman, Don H.
1978   "Ethnomethodology." *The American Sociologist* 13:6–14.
Zimmerman, Don H., and Melvin Pollner
1970   "The everyday world as a phenomenon." Pp. 33–65, in H.
        Pepinsky (ed.), *People and Information.* Elmsford, New York:
        Pergamon.
Zimmerman, Don H., and Candace West
1975   "Sex roles, interruptions, and silences in conversation." Pp.
        105–129, in B. Thorne and N. Henley (eds.), *Language and
        Sex: Difference and Dominance.* Rowley, Massachusetts: New-
        bury House.
Zola, Irving Kenneth
1963   "Problems of communication, diagnosis, and patient care:
        The interplay of patient, physician and clinic organization."
        Journal of Medical Education 38:829–838.
Zola, Irving Kenneth
1966   "Culture and symptoms: An analysis of patients presenting
        complaints." *American Sociological Review* 31:615–630.
Zola, Irving Kenneth
1973   "Pathways to the doctor—from person to patient." *Social Sci-
        ence and Medicine* 7:667–689.

Index